Weight Bias in Health Education

Weight stigma is so pervasive in our culture that it is often unnoticed, along with the harm that it causes. Health care is rife with anti-fat bias and discrimination against fat people, which compromises care and influences the training of new practitioners.

This book explores how this happens and how we can change it. This interdisciplinary volume is grounded in a framework that challenges the dominant discourse that health in fat individuals must be improved through weight loss. The first part explores the negative impacts of bias, discrimination, and other harms by health care providers against fat individuals. The second part addresses how we can "fatten" pedagogy for current and future health care providers, discussing how we can address anti-fat bias in education for health professionals and how alternative frameworks, such as Health at Every Size, can be successfully incorporated into training so that health outcomes for fat people improve.

Examining what works and what fails in teaching health care providers to truly care for the health of fat individuals without further stigmatizing them or harming them, this book is for scholars and practitioners with an interest in fat studies and health education from a range of backgrounds, including medicine, nursing, social work, nutrition, physiotherapy, psychology, sociology, education, and gender studies.

Heather A. Brown is the Assistant Director of the University Writing Center at the A.T. Still University College of Graduate Health Studies. She earned an MTS from Harvard Divinity School and an EdD in Adult and Higher Education from Northern Illinois University. Her research is focused on the connections between weight and learning and how to promote academic achievement in fat women in postsecondary education.

Nancy Ellis-Ordway is a psychotherapist in private practice in Jefferson City, Missouri, with 35 years' experience; she specializes in treating eating disorders, body image issues, stress, anxiety, depression, and relationship issues. She earned a Master of Social Work degree from Washington University and has a PhD in Health Education and Promotion from the University of Missouri.

Routledge Studies in the Sociology of Health and Illness

Weight Bias in Health Education

Critical Perspectives for Pedagogy and Practice

Edited by
Heather A. Brown
Nancy Ellis-Ordway

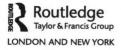

LONDON AND NEW YORK

First published 2021
by Routledge
2 Park Square, Milton Park, Abingdon, Oxon OX14 4RN

and by Routledge
52 Vanderbilt Avenue, New York, NY 10017

Routledge is an imprint of the Taylor & Francis Group, an informa business

British Library Cataloguing-in-Publication Data
A catalogue record for this book is available from the British Library

Library of Congress Cataloging-in-Publication Data
A catalog record has been requested for this book

ISBN: 978-0-367-52230-8 (hbk)
ISBN: 978-1-032-11216-9 (pbk)
ISBN: 978-1-003-05700-0 (ebk)

DOI: 10.4324/9781003057000

Typeset in Goudy
by KnowledgeWorks Global Ltd.

Contents

PART II
Fattening pedagogy 81

Contributors

Roya Amirniroumand is a doctoral student in clinical psychology at Nova Southeastern University. Her research interests include pediatric health disparities, cultural competency among providers, and community-based participatory models of research.

Alex Andrews is a second year Social Work student at Ryerson University, Toronto. They hold a Honours Bachelor of Arts from the University of Toronto. Their research focuses on the intersection of fatness and disability.

Catherine Baker-Pitts holds a PhD and completed post-doctoral training in psychotherapy and psychoanalysis at New York University. Her writing and private practice in New York City focus on gender creativity and body liberation.

Meredith Bessey is PhD student at the University of Guelph, in the Department of Family Relations and Applied Nutrition. She is interested in the transformational possibility of critical, arts-based research to shift thinking about bodies, weight and food within dietetics practice and pedagogy.

Jennifer Renee Blevins holds a PhD in American literature from the University of South Carolina, where she is a Bridge Humanities Postdoctoral Teaching Fellow.

Jennifer Brady is a dietitian and an assistant professor at Mount Saint Vincent University in Halifax, Nova Scotia. Her research interests span critical, feminist perspectives of food, nutrition, eating, bodies, and expertise. She is particularly interested in the history and professionalization of dietetics and its forbearer, home economics, as well as health professionals' roles as advocates in social justice and health equity.

Paula M. Brochu is a social psychologist and associate professor in the Department of Clinical and School Psychology at Nova Southeastern University. Her research examines the processes underlying the expression of weight bias, the consequences of weight bias, and the efficacy of weight bias reduction interventions.

Lisa M. Brownstone is a visiting clinical assistant professor of counseling psychology at the University of Denver's Morgridge College of Education. She completed her PhD in clinical psychology at the University of North Carolina at Chapel Hill, as well as her pre-doctoral clinical internship at the Denver VA Medical Center and post-doctoral fellowship at Eating Disorder Care of

Denver. Her scholarship, clinical work, and teaching focus on disordered eating and body distress, trauma, stigma, psychotherapy, and identity.

Hannah Cory is a registered dietitian and a President's Postdoctoral Fellow at the University of Minnesota. As a clinician she works predominantly with adolescent young people and her research explores how experiences of weight stigma intersect with other forms of oppression for young people of color and in turn, impact chronic disease outcomes.

Joy Cox works for the Office of Diversity and Community Engagement at Rutgers New Jersey Medical School and is a Qualitative Research Fellow at Stanford University School of Medicine. She earned her PhD. in Communication from Rutgers University. Her work focuses on intersectionality addressing race, body size, accessibility, and "health" within the context of body acceptance and fat liberation.

Virginia Dicken-Gracen is a health and psychology educator. She earned her MPH in community health education and MS in applied psychology from Southern Illinois University, Carbondale. She teaches college courses on diversity and inclusion in health care, the psychosocial aspects of health, and the intersections of race, gender, and science at Western Michigan University.

Chelsea D'Silva is a health researcher with background in community health. She is a research associate at the Institute for Better Health, Trillium Health Partners.

Dianne Fierheller has been working with a diverse group of children and families as a pediatric health care social worker since 2004. Dianne is a PhD candidate at McMaster University in the Department of Social Work and an IBH investigator at the Institute for Better Health, Trillium Health Partners. Her current research explores mothering experiences of participating in pediatric weight management programs.

May Friedman's research looks at unstable identities, including bodies that do not conform to traditional racial and national or aesthetic lines. Most recently much of May's research has focused on intersectional approaches to fat studies considering the multiple and fluid experiences of both fat oppression and fat activism. May works at Ryerson University as a faculty member in the School of Social Work and in the Ryerson/York graduate program in communication and culture.

Amanda K. Greene is an Andrew W. Mellon postdoctoral research scholar at Lehigh University. Her scholarship is driven by interdisciplinary approaches to human feeling and embodiment, focusing on how illness, pain, and disability are encountered and "read" in everyday life. She has a PhD in English with a graduate certificate in science, technology, and society from the University of Michigan.

Laura Griffin recently graduated with a Bachelor of Social Work and Health Studies from Ryerson University in Toronto, Ontario. She holds a BA in Sociology and Gender Studies from Memorial University of Newfoundland, in St. John's, Newfoundland.

Christine Heidebrecht is a health researcher with a background in medical anthropology and epidemiology. She is a research associate at the Institute for

Better Health, Trillium Health Partners. Her research interests include health equity, community health, health systems, and program evaluation.

Amanda Hollahan is completing a Bachelor of Social Work from Ryerson University, Toronto. She is interested in examining the intersections of fatness and gender; the impacts of familial and intimate-partner violence; and the ways in which dominant power structures such as Whiteness, sexism, and heteronormativity are enacted through our legal system. Amanda also works with WomenatthecentrE, producing their bi-weekly podcast.

Elizabeth Lanphier is a faculty member in the Ethics Center at Cincinnati Children's Hospital Medical Center, an assistant professor of pediatrics in the University of Cincinnati College of Medicine, and an assistant professor of philosophy at the University of Cincinnati. She work on issues in moral philosophy and clinical ethics from feminist perspectives.

Sara Martel is currently training in psychotherapy and counseling in Toronto, Ontario. She has a PhD in Communication & Culture, and researches and writes about the social, cultural, and political aspects of health and illness.

Sonia Meerai is a full-time PhD student within the Gender, Feminist, and Women Studies Program at York University, Toronto, Ontario. Her commitment within her work is dismantling oppressive practices within mental health and health care systems through her social work practice and in her research.

Rachel Millner is a psychologist, a certified eating disorder specialist and approved supervisor, and a certified body trust provider. In addition to her clinical work, she speaks nationally on weight stigma, anorexia in higher weight bodies, and about her own eating disorder recovery.

Lauren Muhlheim is a psychologist, fellow of the Academy for Eating Disorders, and certified eating disorder specialist and approved supervisor. She directs Eating Disorder Therapy LA in Los Angeles providing evidence-based treatment for eating disorders.

Helia Nabavian is a first-year medical student at the University of Toronto. She has a personal and professional passion for understanding and addressing stigma and health, which she pursues in community organizing and as part of her medical practice.

Alexandria M. Schmidt received her BS in psychology and MS in clinical psychology at the University of Alaska Anchorage. She is pursuing her PhD in clinical psychology at Nova Southeastern University in Ft. Lauderdale, Florida. Her research interests include health behaviors, eating disorders, binge-eating, and consequences of weight bias.

Fady Shanouda is an assistant professor at Carleton University in Ottawa, Ontario. His scholarly contributions lie at the theoretical and pedagogical intersections of disability, mad, and fat Studies and include examinations that surface the interconnections of colonialism, racism, ableism/sanism, and fatphobia.

Ian Zenlea is a pediatric endocrinologist at Trillium Health Partners and a clinician scientist at the Institute for Better Health. Ian's current research focuses on understanding social determinants of health in relation to family and child health.

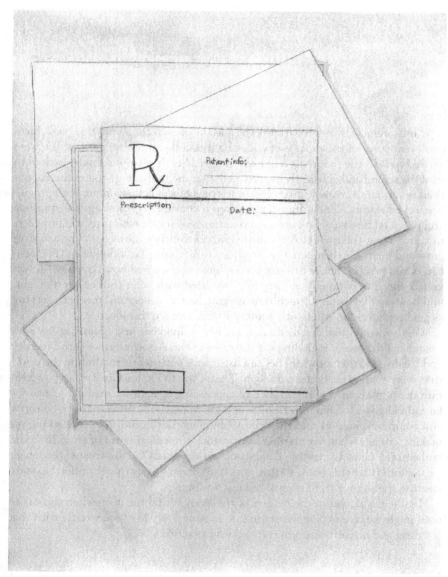

Image courtesy of Genevieve Kirk

Acknowledgements

First and foremost, we wish to thank the authors of each chapter in this book. Each and every stage of the process of collating this collection was exciting! We were excited to read the proposals and excited to read early chapters drafts, excited to read the strong and powerful chapters as they came to fruition, and excited about their potential to create lasting change in the medical field – among both providers and educators. The authors have taken a courageous stand against injustice and provided new ways for current and future health care educators and providers to think about their work. Are they helping or are they harming? How can they grow and change in a system that rewards harm against fat individuals? The educators and practitioners writing in this volume also showed how they have grown and changed over time, how they have wrestled with what they've been taught, and how they've come through that struggle better healers and teachers, serving as guiding lights for others who want and need to take this journey.

We also would like to thank a number of individuals and organizations who influenced this work, including the members of the Association for Size Diversity and Health and the ShowMeTheData listserv for persistently reminding the world that there is another, better paradigm. Thank you to Dr. Joy Cox for her powerful introduction about the importance of continuing to fight for medical justice for fat individuals. Dr. Elizabeth Belasco and Dr. Mary Barile provided both editorial and emotional support and the occasional much need goad to keep working on making change when yet another horror story of medical harm of fat individuals broke in the news. Genevieve Kirk, studio art major at Oberlin, created the image we use for PR for this book, so this work can serve as a new "prescription" to start treating the ills of weight stigma and discrimination.

Finally, thank you to the readers of this book for taking it up when the easier path might be to embrace the status quo in your work. May you wrestle with this learning and may it transform you and your practice.

Preface

How do we reeducate a nation?
Joy Cox

The night came quickly on that day. As I looked around the room, I was the only one left. There was a chill in the air, as it normally was. The screen from my laptop was glaring. The cushion running thin from sitting, I could now start to feel how uncomfortable the "plush" computer chair really was. Knowing this was my last day, I tried to savor the moment. I took a long hard look at the screen as my mind drifted back to the times of vigorous debates, some laughs, and more than often frustration and disenchantment. I knew I was making the right decision to officially walk away from being the all-star, well-informed, Internet fatphobia slayer I believed myself to be. It was not that I no longer believed in the cause; in fact, that may have been the very catalyst for my departure. But it was more so that the education I was attempting to give through hard facts, snarky remarks, and at times ALL CAPS emphasis, was not accomplishing the goals that I had hoped for. This technique for educating did not result in grateful hearts acknowledging facts about how we as a society have been miseducated about fat, fatness, and its implications. It did not convert non-believers into fat accepting enthusiasts who ran home to tell their families about the joy they found in self-acceptance.

Instead, much of the information I provided was met with astonishing push back, dismissal, and at times, insults. I was accused of being a denier of science while the science I was providing was also being denied. To add, I found that even in times of coming out as victor of a discussion or debate, I did not feel like my job as an educator had been fully met. I could celebrate for proving my detractors wrong, but that did not translate into societal behavior change around fat bodies. It did not render modifications to policy and regulations that would allow fat people to be seen as a protected class or ensure that accommodations be provided to us in our workplaces. Nevertheless, I knew there would be great fanfare in my echo chamber of fat liberation. Preaching to the choir is always invigorating as they know when to "amen" a statement and heart react a status that captures the essence of the fat Black experience. Yet still, there was something missing. The question burned down deep in my conscious after every "battle" won or lost. How do we reeducate a nation?

If you are an individual residing in any corner of the United States, you know there is a clear disdain for fat bodies. Fatphobia transcends race, age, gender, and ability. All over this country, fat people are despised by their families and health care professionals alike. They are seen as failures, individuals incapable of harnessing self-control to stop their consumption of "bad" foods through the eyes of society. We are the third wheels of every partnership. The absolute last player to be picked on teams. The narratives written about us are harsh. The stereotypes harsher. Yet, perhaps what is most egregious about these feelings and incorrect assumptions is that they often find their way into the books and publications of what we consider some of the most prestigious facilities in the world.

How can any fat person be assured that they will receive adequate care in facilities with health care workers who have been taught that their size is reflective of the feelings they have about themselves and that they lack willpower to achieve goals that will assist in making them healthy? How much trust should a fat person put into a doctor who repeatedly prescribes weight loss despite their office visit having nothing to do with their weight? With health care's integrity on the line, how is it that the body mass index is still, still seen as measurement of any sort as it relates to health, and why is this "tool" that is now seen as supplemental to health assessments so hard to replace with a different supplement knowing its origination? I have confidence that the research I have reviewed throughout my time studying fatness and health would say that there indeed are replacements and other ways to measure health. Moreover, even the concept of health in and of itself.

As of now and historically, fat liberationists and those who adhere to societal norms around fatness have been on opposite sides of the table exchanging information very much in the same way that I was online. We have debated one another many times over. At times, fat people have seen glimmers of hope in small changes made locally through states as it relates to discrimination practices; the influx of health care workers who align themselves with Health at Every Size (HAES™) principles shows that education is reaching beyond what those in health care have typically been taught, yet that is not enough.

Science that backs principles of fat acceptance, though seen as less, is in no way such. Scholars who study fatness, who arrive at very different conclusions than the running narratives we see in mainstream society, utilize the same methodology and review practices as those who stick to fatphobic interpretations of data. Those who find conclusions within their research that fat does not cause disease or a decreased quality of life collect data in the same ways as it is taught in most academe. Still, there remains opposition to these notions, findings, and meta-analyses. There remains scoffing and opposition when we discuss that weight stigma causes more harm than weight itself (ironically supported by research from the Centers for Disease Control and Prevention).

This ongoing tension is one that is nestled within pedagogy but can also be rooted out by its practice. Within our grasp we have the access AND resources to reeducate this population, which houses the next generation of doctors, nurses, and practitioners, on the importance of shredding stigma around marginalized identities that would impede their care. We educators can put societal change into action by accepting research outcomes with .05 and below p values that suggest there is not a significant difference in mortality between those who are fat and those who are not. Broadening pedagogy around these issues, not restricting its voice, is what is needed to ensure that ethics are upheld. It is what is needed to ensure that the Hippocratic Oath taken by doctors is still valid when they interact with fat patients. Students need to hear the ways that weight stigma limits access to care, causing harm and they need to hear this from people with MDs, DOs, PhDs, and any other entity holding power to speak on these matters.

As many should have expected, my departure from debating in online forums was not the end of my commitment to education in fat acceptance. I sat many nights with tense shoulders and a clinched jaw watching misinformation be spread about my community. Some spread it in ignorance and others with blatant indignation and disregard for my existence on the planet, making my pivot to finding another way to educate of great importance. Utilizing pedagogy as a praxis of activism is not a new concept. For decades some of the most well-known social justice movements in the United States have held teach-ins to educate and equip those interested in fighting for various causes. My position in this was of no difference, as arguably the quest to reeducate the masses about fatness has become a work of activism given the implications of the miseducation that preceded it.

The year is 2017 when I find myself in a unique position to take the education I have utilized and stored in the vessels in my mind to accepting and non-accepting spaces. I begin my practice in teaching with facts, as always, but not with the intent of simply proving detractors wrong. What I have learned in this process is that there will always be detractors. The exhaustion it takes to debate with someone online about a topic they genuinely have no stake in, leaves the one most invested depleted. Instead, I focus on the message and outcome that I seek to achieve by sharing the information I have accumulated. I focus on the change I wish to see in academia and health care. I look members of the crowd in their eyes and challenge them to discount me and my life the way those behind the screen do. Questions are asked and answered. Arguments are made and dispelled. I walk away firm in knowing nothing can be said or done that justifies stripping a person of humanity due to the size of their person. Facts can be debated, but they cannot be replaced. Even if buried, they will eventually bloom again and reveal the beauty of their existence.

As I now stand in solidarity with institutions that use medical education with a restorative justice framework, I have the privilege to speak to doctors about the impact of weight stigma and what can be done to mitigate its use. We speak at length, understanding that health care is not an innocent bystander in regard to fatphobia but a driving force in perpetuating its harm. Through our own experience in the pedagogy of health care, one that includes fat liberation, we inform our practices by redistributing power to those with lived experiences in fat bodies and openly critique the shortcomings of previous research studies and health care practices that have left a stain on ethical care that cannot and should not be washed away.

When medical students enter my classroom to have didactic sessions about weight stigma and health care's role, I am often taken aback at their empathy and care. I also listen to their stories, understanding that they too are coming from experiences slightly different than those of generations before. Some of my students are fat. Some have fat family members. Others have also suffered at the hands of weight stigma, struggling to understand why their existence rendered negative treatment from those whom they had been taught to trust the most. All are looking to be the best version of themselves to give proper care to their patients.

Perhaps this is where the focus should be? Pedagogy is not about the teacher teaching material that aligns with their view. As an educator, I am not interested in creating small versions of myself through my students that they might go about attempting to do their best impersonation of Dr. Cox. No, rather I am simply passing on information with a focus in mind that we can both agree on. I am hoping to share this information with my students and watch it transform into practice in a way that is palatable for them. I need not be seen.

Audre Lorde is lauded and often recited when we speak about the inability of the master's house being dismantled by his own tools. Jane Eliot speaks to the United States' educational system being one of indoctrination as opposed to learning with a freedom to choose. As educators and researchers, our focus should not be to push a narrative, especially if that narrative is contradicted, disputed, and dismantled by empirical evidence that is ethically sound and rooted in equity. The table of education should expand to accommodate others. The conversation should be broadened as a result. A result that, in the end, makes us all better, well-informed participants in the work of equitable care.

When students share stories during sessions that help to illuminate how health care has been a proponent of weight stigma and subpar care as it relates to fat patients based on the information they have received, I see the power of pedagogy at work. I watch as they draw conclusions through their own critical thinking skills to come up with a conclusion based on the information provided them. When we talk solutions for a patient, I watch as they find ways to center the individual's needs first as opposed to what they recommend. They start to speak about the importance of culture and what it would mean to a patient if they were forced to sit out on special events because of restrictive eating plans. They speak candidly about barriers to access in discussions about fitness for patients and why being poor or living in certain neighborhoods make this recommendation obsolete. Lastly, I watch their faces light up when speaking about the impact of genetics and explaining that there is so much more to body size than just eating food and moving the body. They sit as sponges ready to take in information. Some also sit as those who have been waiting to hear that they are just as worthy to receive respect and that their body does not disqualify them from quality care.

It would be a dishonest assessment to say that weight stigma and the miseducation of fat is not a double-edged sword that cuts those who thrust it as well as those who are the intended target. The fallout of this is clear as the body mass index cannot adequately measure the difference between fat and muscle, people in smaller bodies go undiagnosed for problems typically attributed to larger bodies, and those in mental health see an uptick in clients who suffer from conditions like orthorexia. What joy we should feel knowing that there is education out there that can help us in addressing these issues!

Weight Bias in Health Education: Critical Perspectives for Pedagogy and Practice assists us in filling a gap that is needed and necessary medical education and beyond if we position ourselves as educators poised to train the next generation of healers. We do no harm in allowing research to speak for itself. We do no harm in giving a platform to fat Black, Indigenous, disabled, and queer bodies to give accounts of their own lived experiences in health care and the implications of such. This education offers health care professionals a glimpse into the future but also a walk through the past to examine the harm of what has been the traditional way of doing health. It amplifies the silenced voices often drowned out in the numbers of quantitative outcomes and models that focus on majorities when speaking about those marginalized. With a comprehensive coverage of topics that span physical and mental health care, the material between the proceeding pages will show that bodies are complex and cannot be understood through a phobic lens. By broadening our education and the resources we lean on for intelligence, we can expand our reach beyond the choirs who love to hear us preach. In broadening our pedagogy, we only have as Fannie Lou Hamer said, our chains to lose.

1 Introduction

Documented harm: How a misguided paradigm hurts fat people (and everybody else)

Heather A. Brown and Nancy Ellis-Ordway

In just four panels, the cartoon (Deutsch, 2018) encapsulates the issue at the heart of this compilation. In it, a heavy woman sits on a doctor's examination table. She is holding her left arm, which is not attached to her body. She asks for help since her arm has fallen off in the middle of the night for an unknown reason. The doctor looks at the patient:

> DOCTOR: Hmmmm .... First thing, let's get you on a diet.
> PATIENT: A diet? To reconnect my arm?

The patient is frustrated and angry. She demands treatment for the problem for which she is seeking help. The doctor, instead of helping, questions the patient about how much fast food she eats a day. The cartoon ends with the doctor writing her visit notes: "Patient was uncooperative ..." (Deutsch, 2018).

The first time we saw the cartoon, we nodded our heads in recognition of what is, for us and many of the professionals with whom we work, a universal truth. For fat people of all races, genders, and socioeconomic statuses, of all education levels, sexual orientations, or religious affiliations, doctors often are unhelpful (at best) or cruel (at worst)—if fat individuals engage with them at all. For those with multiple marginalized identities, the harm they experience at the hands of medical professionals can be even worse; they face the stigma of not only their race, their gender, their income levels, their (dis)ability, and/or their queerness, but also their weight (Cox, 2020; Ellis-Ordway, 2019; Farrell, 2011; Greenhalgh, 2015; Hebl et al., 2003; Lind, 2020; Oliver, 2006a; Rinaldi et al., 2020; Robinson, 2020; Strings, 2019).

The oath that health care providers take is one that requires them to avoid malfeasance, or do no harm, yet the health care field is rife with harmful anti-fat bias and discrimination against fat people (Schwartz et al., 2003; Teachman & Brownell, 2001). More than 50% of doctors describe their fat patients as ugly, lazy, noncompliant, weak-willed, dishonest, and unintelligent (Campbell et al., 2000; Ferrante et al., 2009; Fogelman et al., 2002; Foster et al., 2003; Hebl & Xu, 2001; Huizinga et al., 2009; Price et al., 1987; Puhl & Heuer, 2009). Among nurses, 24% admit to being repulsed by fat patients, preferring not to care for them (Brown, 2006; Puhl & Brownell, 2001). Future health care providers exhibit similar beliefs.

DOI: 10.4324/9781003057000-1

Medical students and students in other health care fields describe fat people as unpleasant, sloppy, and lacking in self-control (Berryman et al., 2006; Blumberg & Mellis, 1985; Keane, 1990; Persky & Eccleston, 2011; Puhl et al., 2009; Wigton & McGaghie, 2001).

And fat individuals know their health care providers are biased against them (Bertakis & Azari, 2005; Wadden et al., 2000). For example, nearly 70% of fat women have reported experiencing bias from a doctor (Puhl & Brownell, 2006). As a result, many fat patients avoid seeking preventative care, leading to poorer health outcomes than non-fat individuals with similar illnesses (Amy et al., 2006).

The prevalence of anti-fat bias and discrimination among health care providers and the consequences of that bias are so problematic that organizations like the Rudd Center for Food Policy and Obesity have developed a series of online learning modules to help providers learn about the negative effects of weight bias on health and on fat people's access to health care. Yet, this work is still situated within a framework arguing that health is improved through weight loss. This dominant "obesity" paradigm is still problematic because a focus on improving health through weight loss is not only counterproductive but also highly damaging.

A failed intervention

Recommendations for weight loss are common in medical treatment but they cannot be considered evidence-based. In 1959, Stunkard and McLaren-Hume analyzed the ubiquitous lack of success in weight loss attempts and concluded that weight-loss treatments were potentially dangerous and should be undertaken only rarely and then with caution. In the six decades since, a large and growing body of research continues to support the consistent failure of attempts to lose weight, by any method.

The human body will adapt metabolically to restricted intake (Leibel et al., 1995; Ochner et al., 2015). Hunger increases in response to decreased energy intake, overwhelming determination and will power (Macpherson-Sánchez, 2015). When followed for 2 years or more, the vast majority, 95% or more, of dieters will regain the weight they lost—and sometimes more (Bacon & Aphramor, 2011; Fildes et al., 2015; Hunger et al., 2020; Tomiyama et al., 2013; Tylka et al., 2014). In fact, restrictive eating for weight control is a robust predictor of weight *gain* (Bacon & Aphramor, 2011; Bacon et al., 2005; Mann et al., 2007).

"The benefits of dieting are simply too small and the potential harms of dieting are too large for it to be recommended as a safe and effective treatment for obesity" (Mann et al., 2007, p. 230). Overwhelming evidence and vast personal experience contradict the prevailing idea that body size is under the control of the individual. If weight is considered a risk factor, it is a non-modifiable one, given the failure of interventions to change it.

The prevailing focus on weight loss as helpful is largely driven by financial interests (Oliver, 2006b). As of 2019, the diet industry in the United States was worth more than $72 billion (Marketdata LLC, 2019). That kind of money has far-reaching influence, often obscuring evidence-based approaches to treatment.

Conflating weight and health

The connections between weight and health are complex even though the connection between being fat and having poor health is portrayed in the media and, indeed, in many doctor's offices as clear cut, proven, and undeniable; perhaps the only clear connection in the literature is that weight is not a trustworthy proxy for health. The belief that higher body weight causes disease relies on correlational data while ignoring other variables, such as health behaviors, weight stigma, and social determinants (Bacon & Aphramor, 2011; Calogero et al., 2018). The widely held assumption that weight loss equals improved health is not well supported by evidence. In some cases, the relationship between higher weight and poor health is confounded by other factors that may be driving both (Hunger et al., 2020). For instance, insulin resistance leads to both diabetes and weight gain. A meta-analysis of weight loss studies that followed participants for 1 year found minimal to no improvements in health outcomes related to weight loss (Tomiyama et al., 2013). Longer-term interventions found even weaker evidence supporting health benefits from weight loss (Hunger et al., 2020), and, in some studies, higher body weights are actually associated with a concept called the "obesity paradox," in which individuals who are classified as "overweight" or "obese" see health protections during certain chronic illness as opposed to their weight being harmful to their health (Cao et al., 2012; Kalantar-Zadeh et al., 2004; Niedziela et al., 2014; Padwal et al., 2014; Schmidt & Salahudeen, 2007; Sharma et al., 2015; Veronese et al., 2015; Wang et al., 2016). Moreover, if one uses the arbitrary categories of the body mass index (BMI), the actual mortality rates for the "overweight" group is lower than for the "normal" category (Flegal et al., 2013; O'Hara & Taylor, 2018).

BMI is easy to use, requiring only a scale and measurement of height. BMI is the primary classification system used to drive discussions between doctor and patient about health. BMI does not measure health or behaviors; however, healthy behaviors are correlated with improved health across BMI categories. Matheson et al. (2012) studied the association between mortality and lifestyle habits (specifically, not smoking, eating at least five fruits and vegetables daily, physical activity, and moderate alcohol intake) and found increasing health benefits with increased healthy behaviors for people of all sizes, including those classified as "normal" weight under BMI. When health is evaluated by BMI, slender people (and their doctors) may assume they are healthy and have no need to engage in health promoting behaviors. Health improvements in people pursuing weight loss may be due to changes in behavior but are assumed to be caused by the weight loss (Tomiyama et al., 2013). The almost inevitable weight regain is perceived as "failure," resulting in abandonment of the health-promoting behaviors (Vartanian & Shaprow, 2008). Meanwhile, long-term improvements in health related to weight loss could only be evaluated accurately by comparing always-thin people to previously-fat-and-now-thin people, which is not possible when we do not have a large representative group of previously fat people who have remained thin for several years.

Using the BMI as a measure of cardiometabolic health risks misclassifying almost a quarter of the population as unhealthy simply based on weight and height. Almost half of those considered "overweight," 29% of those in the "obese" and 16% of those in "obesity class II and III," are metabolically healthy, while 30% of those in the "normal" category are metabolically unhealthy (Tomiyama et al., 2016). Meanwhile, cardiorespiratory fitness may be a better predictor of mortality than BMI but when the success of health interventions is evaluated only by weight loss, improved fitness is undervalued (Bombak, 2014).

Moreover, BMI is a racist tool based on northern European body standards from a specific historical point in time; as a result, BMI has often been used to disparage other racial and ethnic communities that had naturally larger bodies (Strings, 2019). Asian populations, traditionally smaller than their northern European counterparts, on the other hand, are given an even lower BMI cut-off point for what counts as "obesity" (Hood et al., 2019; Misra & Dhurandhar, 2019). For individuals who are not White, "[t]he fear and shame of living in a fat body come dressed in the same racist, fatphobic bullshit the West has been selling for centuries" (Cox, 2020, pp. 19–20). In fact, many of the health concerns commonly correlated with high BMI also can be correlated with surviving systemic racism (Chambers et al., 2004; Dougherty et al., 2020; Gee et al., 2008; Mwendwa et al., 2011).

LGBTQ+ individuals face additional challenges related to BMI. For example, there is current debate about whether transgender individuals with high BMI should be allowed to have gender-confirmation surgery. Some researchers (see Martinson et al., 2020) argue that transgender individuals with high BMIs present too great a risk during the surgical procedure to be allowed to access this living saving surgery. Others argue that BMI prerequisites are not only not evidence-based (Brownstone et al., 2020) but also that there is no evidence that transgender individuals with high BMIs who do have surgery have higher levels of complications than those with lower BMIs (Rothenberg et al., 2019). Martinson et al. (2020), interestingly, found that efforts at weight loss prior to gender-affirming surgery were "unsuccessful" even among "individuals who would be predicted to be motivated" (p. 6). This "fact" seems particularly cruel when recent research shows that the rate of suicide attempts among transgender individuals decreases markedly following gender-affirming surgery (Bränström & Pachankis, 2020).

Many of the physical maladies commonly considered to be caused by weight may, in fact, be caused by weight-cycling, also known as "yo-yo dieting." Repeated weight fluctuations may stress the cardiometabolic systems, leading to increased morbidity and mortality (Bangalore et al., 2017; Montani et al., 2015.) Weight cycling has been linked to greater emotional distress, loss of lean muscle mass, reduced metabolic energy expenditure, and increased risk of osteoporotic fractures, gall stones, hypertension, chronic inflammation, and some forms of cancer. A focus on weight loss also increases weight stigma, which is also associated with poorer health outcomes (Bombak, 2014; Muennig et al., 2008; Tylka et al., 2014).

Indeed, it is impossible and should be unethical to evaluate the relationship between health and weight without also considering the effects of weight stigma in medical treatment. Larger people may avoid seeking health care if they have been shamed at the doctor's office, thus delaying diagnosis and treatment (Amy et al., 2006; Aphramor, 2012; Pausé, 2017). This avoidance is understandable, given the documented weight bias among health professionals (Phelan et al., 2014) but it is not possible to measure fully the impact this has on long-term health outcomes.

An alternative approach

A weight-loss first approach to health care provision is highly problematic. And although it was challenging to find medical doctors and nurses to write for this book since many are invested in the weight-loss first approach and are compensated for it by insurance companies now that "obesity" is classified as a disease (Kyle et al. 2016), many dieticians, social workers, nutritionists, psychologists, and therapists as well as educators of future health care professionals and even a few doctors themselves recognize the need for a new paradigm: "For starters, we need a new approach, founded on respect and dignity for patients" (Prologo, 2020, para. 26).

Fat Studies, as a field and as a theoretical framework, offers an alternative. Rothblum and Solovay (2009) defined the discipline as

> an interdisciplinary field of scholarship marked by an aggressive, consistent, rigorous critique of the negative assumptions, stereotypes, and stigma placed on fat and the fat body. The field of Fat Studies invites scholars to pause, interrupt the everyday thinking about fat (or failure to think), and do something daring and bold. (p. 2)

Fat Studies is a field that approaches "the construction of fat and fatness with a critical methodology—the same sort of progressive, systematic academic rigor with which we approach negative attitudes and stereotypes about women, queer people, and racial groups" (Rothblum & Solovay, 2009, p. 2). Moreover, Fat Studies is a field focused on the lived experience of real people. Placing the experiences of the fat individual at the heart of research and practice is vitally important because research that utilizes the dominant medical paradigm often does not address fat individuals as real, self-defining people, instead treating them as either statistics or tissue to be manipulated and changed for their own good.

Finally, Fat Studies argues that the dominant discourse establishing "obesity" as a medical problem or a disease must be problematized. Weight is never just a medical issue to be addressed using medical solutions; it is more complex than that. Issues of health and disease in fat individuals are often conflated with issues of morality. "When we define fatness as a disease we are acting within powerful social boundaries which control what we believe to be right and appropriate, or shameful and abnormal" (Cooper, 1998, p. 71). This is especially true when fatness is presented as a temporary, fixable "problem" that is wholly under the control of the individual (Cooper, 1998). Under such a framing, the fat individual becomes a pariah, responsible for all the hate and bias aimed at them, issues that would go away if only the fat person would just lose weight. "Belief in a 'cure' also masks that hatred. It is not possible to hate a group of people for our own good. Medicalization actually helps categorize fat people as social untouchables" (Wann, 2009, p. xiv). As social untouchables responsible for their own stigmatization, fat individuals become unworthy of the rights of "normal" citizens, including access to unbiased and supportive health care that is not focused on weight loss as the cure for each and every ailment.

This collection, grounded in Fat Studies, provides a start for that new paradigm called for above. It explores the negative impacts of bias, discrimination, and other harms by health care providers against fat individuals. It asks—and answers— how we can "fatten" pedagogy for current and future health care providers. How can we address anti-fat bias in the seminal stages of medical education? How can alternative frameworks, such as Health at Every Size™, be successfully incorporated into training new doctors, nurses, and other medical professionals, including physical therapists, dietitians, social workers, etc.? What works and what fails in teaching health care providers to truly care for the health of fat individuals without further stigmatizing them or harming them?

Conclusion

This book is not intended for those who are well-versed in Fat Studies, fat acceptance, or fat liberation. Rather, it serves more as an entry point for health care professionals and students who are seeking a way to better care for the fat individuals with whom they interact. This is one reason why some of the authors will use the word "fat" to describe individuals; these authors are working with the word as an unstigmatized and reclaimed adjective; other authors, who work in certain contexts, will still use words like "overweight" or "obese." Even though these terms are used widely, the term "overweight" implies that there is a proper weight to be and that any deviation is unacceptable, while "obese" implies medical pathology. In this collection, outside of direct quotes from other sources, these words will be in "scare quotes" to indicate the problematic political nature of the terms. An additional note about language: the dominant paradigm that pathologizes larger bodies and focuses on weight loss as an intervention is referred to as "weight-normative" or "weight-loss centered" or "weight-loss first" with alternative approaches referred to as "weight-inclusive" or "weight-neutral."

Regardless of language, all chapter authors were encouraged to explore the undisputed fact that human health is complex and that practices in the education of current and future health care providers tend to over-simplify the connections (or lack thereof) between weight and health. Chapter authors took as their core guidance the need for evidence-based medical care of fat individuals and the necessity for current and future health care providers to receive the education needed to better care for fat individuals as real, whole people, not just adipose tissue to be eradicated. As a result, you hold in your hands not just another book cataloguing the failures of dominant medical discourse on "obesity," but rather real solutions that fatten pedagogy so that current and future health care providers can help rather than harm.

References

Amy, N. K., Aalborg, A., Lyons, P., & Keranen, L. (2006). Barriers to routine gynecological cancer screening for White and African-American obese women. *International Journal of Obesity, 30*(1), 147–155. https://doi.org/10.1038/sj.ijo.0803105

Aphramor, L. (2012). The impact of a weight-centred treatment approach on women's health and health-seeking behaviours. *Journal of Critical Dietetics, 1*(2), 3–12.

Bacon, L., & Aphramor, L. (2011). Weight science: Evaluating the evidence for a paradigm shift. *Nutrition Journal, 10*(1), 9. https://doi.org/10.1186/1475-2891-10-9

Bacon, L., Stern, J. S., Van Loan, M. D., & Keim, N. L. (2005). Size acceptance and intuitive eating improve health for obese, female chronic dieters. *Journal of the American Dietetic Association, 105*(6), 929–936.

Bangalore, S., Fayyad, R., Laskey, R., DeMicco, D. A., Messerli, F. H., & Waters, D. D. (2017). Body-weight fluctuations and outcomes in coronary disease. *New England Journal of Medicine, 376*(14), 1332–1340.

Berryman, D. E., Dubale, G. M., Manchester, D. S., & Mittelstaedt, R. (2006). Dietetics students possess negative attitudes toward obesity similar to nondietetics students. *Journal of the American Dietetic Association, 106*(10), 1678–1682.

Bertakis, K. D., & Azari, R. (2005). The impact of obesity on primary care visits. *Obesity Research, 13*(9), 1615–1623. https://doi.org/10.1038/oby.2005.198

Blumberg, P., & Mellis, L. P. (1985). Medical students' attitudes toward the obese and the morbidly obese. *International Journal of Eating Disorders, 4*(2), 169–175. https://doi.org/10.1002/1098-108X(198505)4:2%3C169::AID-EAT2260040204%3E3.0.CO;2-F

Bombak, A. (2014). Obesity, Health at Every Size, and public health policy. *American Journal of Public Health, 104*(2), e60–e67. https://aiph.aphapublications.org/doi/abs/10.2105/AJPH.2013.301486

Bränström, R., & Pachankis, J. E. (2020). Reduction in mental health treatment utilization among transgender individuals after gender-affirming surgeries: A total population study. *American Journal of Psychiatry, 177*(8), 727–734. https://doi.org/10.1176/appi.ajp.2019.19010080

Brown, I. (2006). Nurses' attitudes towards adult patients who are obese: Literature review. *Journal of Advanced Nursing, 53*(2), 221–232.

Brownstone, L. M., DeRieux, J., Kelly, D. A., Sumlin, L. J., & Gaudiani, J. L. (2020). Body mass index requirements for gender-affirming surgeries are not empirically based. *Transgender health*. Advance online publication. https://doi.org/10.1089/trgh.2020.0068

Calogero, R. M., Tylka, T. L., Mensinger, J. L., Meadows, A., & Daníelsdóttir, S. (2018). Recognizing the fundamental right to be fat: A weight-inclusive approach to size acceptance and healing from sizeism. *Women & Therapy, 42*(1–2), 22–44. https://doi.org/10.1080/02703149.2018.1524067

Campbell, K., Engel, H., Timperio, A., Cooper, C., & Crawford, D. (2000). Obesity management: Australian general practitioners' attitudes and practices. *Obesity Research, 8*(6), 459–466. https://doi.org/10.1038/oby.2000.57

Cao, C., Wang, R., Wang, J., Bunjhoo, H., Xu, Y., & Xiong, W. (2012). Body mass index and mortality in chronic obstructive pulmonary disease: A meta-analysis. *PloS One*, 7(8), e43892. https://doi.org/10.1371/journal.pone.0043892

Chambers, E. C., Tull, E. S., Fraser, H. S., Mutunhu, N. R., Sobers, N., & Niles, E. (2004). The relationship of internalized racism to body fat distribution and insulin resistance among African adolescent youth. *Journal of the National Medical Association*, 96(12), 1594–1598.

Cooper, C. (1998). *Fat and proud: The politics of size*. Women's Press Ltd.

Cox, J. A. R. (2020). *Fat girls in Black bodies: Creating communities of our own*. North Atlantic Books.

Deutsch, B. (2018, October 27). *Doctors and fat patients*. Ampersand: Political cartoons by Barry Deutsch. http://leftycartoons.com/2018/10/27/fat-people-and-doctors/

Dougherty, G. B., Golden, S. H., Gross, A. L., Colantuoni, E., & Dean, L. T. (2020). Measuring structural racism and its association with BMI. *American Journal of Preventive Medicine*, 59(4), 530–537. https://doi.org/10.1016/j.amepre.2020.05.019

Ellis-Ordway, N. (2019). *Thrive at any weight: Eating to nourish body, soul, and self-esteem*. Praeger.

Farrell, A. E. (2011). *Fat shame: Stigma and the fat body in American culture*. New York University Press.

Ferrante, J. M., Piasecki, A. K., Ohman-Strickland, P. A., & Crabtree, B. F. (2009). Family physicians' practices and attitudes regarding care of extremely obese patients. *Obesity*, 17(9), 1710–1716. https://doi.org/10.1038/oby.2009.62

Fildes, A., Charlton, J., Rudisill, C., Littlejohns, P., Prevost, A. T., & Gulliford, M. C. (2015). Probability of an obese person attaining normal body weight: Cohort study using electronic health records. *American Journal of Public Health*, 105(9). https://doi.org/10.2105/ajph.2015.302773

Flegal, K. M., Kit, B. K., Orpana, H., & Graubard, B. I. (2013). Association of all-cause mortality with overweight and obesity using standard body mass index categories: A systematic review and meta-analysis. *JAMA*, 309(1), 71–82. https://10.1001/jama.2012.113905

Fogelman, Y., Vinker, S., Lachter, J., Biderman, A., Itzhak, B., & Kitai, E. (2002). Managing obesity: A survey of attitudes and practices among Israeli primary care physicians. *International Journal of Obesity and Related Metabolic Disorders*, 26(10), 1393–1397. https://doi.org/10.1038/sj.ijo.0802063

Foster, G. D., Wadden, T. A., Makris, A. P., Davidson, D., Sanderson, R. S., Allison, D. B., & Kessler, A. (2003). Primary care physicians' attitudes about obesity and its treatment. *Obesity Research*, 11(10), 1168–1177. https://doi.org/10.1038/oby.2003.161

Gee, G. C., Ro, A., Gavin, A., & Takeuchi, D. T. (2008). Disentangling the effects of racial and weight discrimination on body mass index and obesity among Asian Americans. *American Journal of Public Health*, 98(3), 493–500. https://doi.org/10.2105/AJPH.2007.114025

Greenhalgh, S. (2015). *Fat-talk nation: The human costs of America's war on fat*. Cornell University Press.

Hebl, M. R., & Xu, J. (2001). Weighing the care: Physicians' reactions to the size of a patient. *International Journal of Obesity*, 25(8), 1246–1252. https://doi.org/10.1038/sj.ijo.0801681

Hebl, M. R., Xu, J., & Mason, M. F. (2003). Weighing the care: Patients' perceptions of physician care as a function of gender and weight. *International Journal of Obesity*, 27(2), 269–275. https://doi.org/10.1038/sj.ijo.802231

Hood, K., Ashcraft, J., Watts, K., Hong, S., Choi, W., Heymsfield, S. B., Gautam, R. K., & Thomas, D. (2019). Allometric scaling of weight to height and resulting body mass index thresholds in two Asian populations. *Nutrition & Diabetes, 9*(1), 1–7. https://doi.org/10.1038/s41387-018-0068-3

Huizinga, M. M., Cooper, L. A., Bleich, S. N., Clark, J. M., & Beach, M. C. (2009). Physician respect for patients with obesity. *Journal of General Internal Medicine, 24*(11), 1236–1239. https://doi.org/10.1007/s11606-009-1104-8

Hunger, J. M., Smith, J. P., & Tomiyama, A. J. (2020). An evidence-based rationale for adopting weight-inclusive health policy. *Social Issues and Policy Review, 14*(1), 73–107. https://doi.org/10.1111/sipr.12062

Kalantar-Zadeh, K., Block, G., Horwich, T., & Fonarow, G. C. (2004). Reverse epidemiology of conventional cardiovascular risk factors in patients with chronic heart failure. *Journal of the American College of Cardiology, 43*(8), 1439–1444. https://doi.org/10.1016/j.jacc.2003.11.039

Keane, R. M. (1990). Contemporary beliefs about mental illness among medical students: Implications for education and practice. *Academic Psychiatry, 14*(3), 172–177. https://doi.org/10.1007/BF03341291

Kyle, T. K., Dhurandhar, E. J., & Allison, D. B. (2016). Regarding obesity as a disease: Evolving policies and their implications. *Endocrinology and Metabolism Clinics of North America, 45*(3), 511–520. https://doi.org/10.1016/j.ecl.2016.04.004

Leibel, R. L., Rosenbaum, M., & Hirsch, J. (1995). Changes in energy expenditure resulting from altered body weight. *New England Journal of Medicine, 332*(10), 621–628. https://doi.org/10.1056/nejm199503093321001

Lind, E. R. M. (2020). Queering fat activism: A study in Whiteness. In M. Friedman, C. Rice, & J. Rinaldi (Eds.), *Thickening fat: Fat bodies, intersectionality, and social justice* (pp. 183–193). Routledge.

Macpherson-Sánchez, A. E. (2015). Integrating fundamental concepts of obesity and eating disorders: Implications for the obesity epidemic. *American Journal of Public Health, 105*(4). https://doi.org/10.2105/ajph.2014.302507

Mann, T., Tomiyama, A. J., Westling, E., Lew, A.-M., Samuels, B., & Chatman, J. (2007). Medicare's search for effective obesity treatments: Diets are not the answer. *American Psychologist, 62*(3). 220–233. https://doi.org/10.1037/0003-066X.62.3.220

Marketdata, L. L. C. (2019). *The U.S. weight loss and diet control market: A market research analysis* (15th ed.). Author.

Martinson, T. G., Ramachandran, S., Lindner, R., Reisman, T., & Safer, J. D. (2020). High body mass index is a significant barrier to gender-confirmation surgery for transgender and gender-nonbinary individuals. *Endocrine Practice, 26*(1), 6–15. https://doi.org/10.4158/EP-2019-0345

Matheson, E. M., King, D. E., & Everett, C. J. (2012). Healthy lifestyle habits and mortality in overweight and obese individuals. *Journal of the American Board of Family Medicine, 25*(1), 9–15. https://doi.org/10.3122/jabfm.2012.01.110164

Misra, A., & Dhurandhar, N. V. (2019). Current formula for calculating body mass index is applicable to Asian populations. *Nutrition & Diabetes, 9*(3). https://doi.org/10.1038/s41387-018-0070-9

Montani, J., Schutz, Y., & Dulloo, A. G. (2015). Dieting and weight cycling as risk factors for cardiometabolic diseases: Who is really at risk? *Obesity Reviews, 16*, 7–18. https://doi.org/10.1111/obr.12251

Muennig, P., Jia, H., Lee, R., & Lubetkin, E. (2008). I think therefore I am: Perceived ideal weight as a determinant of health. *American Journal of Public Health, 98*(3), 501–506. https://ajph.aphapublications.org/doi/abs/10.2105/AJPH.2007.114769

Mwendwa, D. T., Gholson, G., Sims, R. C., Levy, S. A., Ali, M., Harrell, C. J., Callender, C. O., & Campbell, A. L. Jr (2011). Coping with perceived racism: A significant factor in the development of obesity in African American women? *Journal of the National Medical Association, 103*(7), 602–608. https://doi.org/10.1016/S0027-9684(15)30386-2

Niedziela, J., Hudzik, B., Niedziela, N., Gąsior, M., Gierlotka, M., Wasilewski, J., Myrda, K., Lekston, A., Poloński, L., & Rozentryt, P. (2014). The obesity paradox in acute coronary syndrome: A meta-analysis. *European Journal of Epidemiology, 29*(11), 801–12. https://doi.org/10.1007/s10654-014-9961-9

O'Hara, L., & Taylor, J. (2018). What's wrong with the "war on obesity?" A narrative review of the weight-centered health paradigm and development of the 3C framework to build critical competency for a paradigm shift. *SAGE Open, 8*(2), 215824401877288. https://doi.org/10.1177/2158244018772888

Ochner, C. N., Tsai, A. G., Kushner, R. F., & Wadden, T. A. (2015). Treating obesity seriously: When recommendations for lifestyle change confront biological adaptations. *The Lancet Diabetes & Endocrinology, 3*(4), 232–234. https://doi.org/10.1016/S2213-8587(15)00009-1

Oliver, J. E. (2006a). *Fat politics: The real story behind America's obesity epidemic.* Oxford University Press.

Oliver, J. E. (2006b). The politics of pathology: How obesity became an epidemic disease. *Perspectives in Biology and Medicine, 49*(4), 611–627. https://doi.org/10.1353/pbm.2006.0062

Padwal, R., McAlister, F., Mcmurray, J., Cowie, M., Rich, M., Pocock, S., Swedberg, K., Maggioni, A., Gamble, G., Ariti, C., Earle, N., Whalley, G., Poppe, K., Doughty, R., & Bayes-Genis, A. (2014). The obesity paradox in heart failure patients with preserved versus reduced ejection fraction: A meta-analysis of individual patient data. *International Journal of Obesity, 38*, 1110–1114. https://doi.org/10.1038/ijo.2013.203

Pausé, C. (2017). Borderline: The ethics of fat stigma in public health. *The Journal of Law, Medicine & Ethics, 45*(4), 510–517. https://doi.org/10.1177/1073110517750585

Persky, S., & Eccleston, C. P. (2011). Medical student bias and care recommendations for an obese versus non-obese virtual patient. *International Journal of Obesity, 35*(5), 728–735. https://doi.org/10.1038/ijo.2010.173

Phelan, S. M., Dovidio, J. F., Puhl, R. M., Burgess, D. J., Nelson, D. B., Yeazel, M. W., Hardeman, R., Perry, S., & Van Ryn, M. (2014). Implicit and explicit weight bias in a national sample of 4,732 medical students: The medical student CHANGES study. *Obesity, 22*(4), 1201–1208. https://doi.org/10.1002/oby.20687

Price, J. H., Desmond, S. M., Krol, R. A., Snyder, F. F., & O'Connell, J. K. (1987). Family practice physicians' beliefs, attitudes, and practices regarding obesity. *American Journal of Preventive Medicine, 3*(6), 339–345. https://doi.org/10.1016/S0749-3797(18)31234-0

Prologo, J. D. (2020, September 8). *A doctor's open apology to those fighting overweight and obesity.* The Conversation. https://theconversation.com/a-doctors-open-apology-to-those-fighting-overweight-and-obesity-145017?fbclid=IwAR2JE4aGYja2owGnlcwMGuEahwP3ZOcMokZNe3dsgGkS3ZBYDlJryJxV63g

Puhl, R. M., & Brownell, K. D. (2006). Confronting and coping with weight stigma: An investigation of overweight and obese adults. *Obesity, 14*(10), 1802–1815. https://doi.org/10.1038/oby.2006.208

Puhl, R. M., & Heuer, C. A. (2009). The stigma of obesity: A review and update. *Obesity, 17*(5), 941–964. https://doi.org/10.1038/oby.2008.636

Puhl, R., & Brownell, K. D. (2001). Bias, discrimination, and obesity. *Obesity Research, 9*(12), 788–805. https://doi.org/10.1038/oby.2001.108

Puhl, R., Wharton, C., & Heuer, C. (2009). Weight bias among dietetics students: Implications for treatment practices. *Journal of the American Dietetic Association, 109*(3), 438–444. https://doi.org/10.1016/j.jada.2008.11.034

Rinaldi, J., Rice, C., & Friedman, M. (2020). Introduction. In M. Friedman, C. Rice, & J. Rinaldi (Eds.), *Thickening fat: Fat bodies, intersectionality, and social justice* (pp. 15–28). Routledge.

Robinson, M. (2020). The big colonial bones of indigenous North America's "obesity epidemic." In M. Friedman, C. Rice, & J. Rinaldi (Eds.), *Thickening fat: Fat bodies, intersectionality, and social justice* (pp. 183–193). Routledge.

Rothblum, E. D., & Solovay, S. (Eds.). (2009). *The fat studies reader.* New York University Press.

Rothenberg, K. A., Gologorsky, R. C., Hojilla, J. C., & Yokoo, K. M. (2019). Obesity is not associated with complications or revisions after gender-affirming mastectomy in transgender patients. *Journal of the American College of Surgeons, 229*(4), S225. https://doi.org/10.1016/j.jamcollsurg.2019.08.494

Schmidt, D. S., & Salahudeen, A. K. (2007). Obesity-survival paradox-still a controversy? *Seminars in Dialysis, 20*(6), 486–492. https://doi.org/10.1111/j.1525-139X.2007.00349.x

Schwartz, M. B., Chambliss, H. O. N., Brownell, K. D., Blair, S. N., & Billington, C. (2003). Weight bias among health professionals specializing in obesity. *Obesity Research, 11*(9), 1033–1039. https://doi.org/10.1038/oby.2003.142

Sharma, A., Lavie, C. J., Borer, J. S., Vallakati, A., Goel, S., Lopez-Jimenez, F., Arbab-Zadeh, A., Mukherjee, D., & Lazar, J. M. (2015). Meta-analysis of the relation of body mass index to all-cause and cardiovascular mortality and hospitalization in patients with chronic heart failure. *The American Journal of Cardiology, 115*(10), 1428–1434. https://doi.org/10.1016/j.amjcard.2015.02.024

Strings, S. (2019). *Fearing the Black body: The racial origins of fat phobia.* New York University Press.

Stunkard, A., & McLaren-Hume, M. (1959). The results of treatment for obesity: A review of the literature and report of a series. *AMA Archives of Internal Medicine, 103*(1), 79–85.

Teachman, B. A., & Brownell, K. D. (2001). Implicit anti-fat bias among health professionals: Is anyone immune? *International Journal of Obesity, 25*(10), 1525–1531. https://doi.org/10.1038/sj.ijo.0801745

Tomiyama, A. J., Ahlstrom, B., & Mann, T. (2013). Long-term effects of dieting: Is weight loss related to health? *Social and Personality Psychology Compass, 7*(12), 861–877. https://doi.org/10.1111/spc3.12076

Tomiyama, A. J., Hunger, J. M., Nguyen-Cuu, J., & Wells, C. (2016). Misclassification of cardiometabolic health when using body mass index categories in NHANES 2005–2012. *International Journal of Obesity, 40*(5), 883–886. https://doi.org/10.1038/ijo.2016.17

Tylka, T. L., Annunziato, R. A., Burgard, D., Daníelsdóttir, S., Shuman, E., Davis, C., & Calogero, R. M. (2014). The weight-inclusive versus weight-normative approach to health: Evaluating the evidence for prioritizing well-being over weight loss. *Journal of Obesity, 2014*, Article 983495. https://doi.org/10.1155/2014/983495

Vartanian, L. R., & Shaprow, J. G. (2008). Effects of weight stigma on exercise motivation and behavior: A preliminary investigation among college-aged females. *Journal of Health Psychology, 13*(1), 131–138. https://doi.org/10.1177%2F1359105307084318

Veronese, N., Cereda, E., Solmi, M., Fowler, S. A., Manzato, E., Maggi, S., Manu, P., Abe, E., Hayashi, K., Allard, J. P., Arendt, B. M., Beck, A., Chan, M., Audrey, Y. J., Lin, W. Y., Hsu, H. S., Lin, C. C., Diekmann, R., Kimyagarov, S., ... Correll, C. U. (2015).

Inverse relationship between body mass index and mortality in older nursing home residents: A meta-analysis of 19,538 elderly subjects. *Obesity Reviews, 16*(11), 1001–1015. https://doi.org/10.1111/obr.12309

Wadden, T. A., Anderson, D. A., Foster, G. D., Bennett, A., Steinberg, C., & Sarwer, D. B. (2000). Obese women's perceptions of their physicians' weight management attitudes and practices. *Archives of Family Medicine, 9*(9), 854.

Wang, L., Liu, W., He, X., Chen, Y., Lu, J., Liu, K., Cao, K., & Yin, P. (2016). Association of overweight and obesity with patient mortality after acute myocardial infarction: A meta-analysis of prospective studies. *International Journal of Obesity, 40*(2), 220–228. https://doi.org/10.1038/ijo.2015.176

Wann, M. (2009). Foreward: Fat studies: An invitation to revolution. In E. Rothblum & S. Solovay (Eds.), *The fat studies reader*. New York University Press.

Wigton, R. S., & McGaghie, W. C. (2001). The effect of obesity on medical students' approach to patients with abdominal pain. *Journal of General Internal Medicine, 16*(4), 262–265. https://doi.org/10.1046/j.1525-1497.2001.016004262.x

Part I

When healers cause harm

Introduction
Nancy Ellis-Ordway

No one enters a medical field with the intention of causing harm, but sometimes they do. Weight stigma and anti-fat bias are so common in our culture as to be unremarkable, and healers are not immune to the effects. Even when we are aware of the harm caused by a weight-centric paradigm, specific examples can slip by us if we are not vigilant.

Confirmation bias is the tendency to pay attention to information that agrees with what we already believe and to discount new material that disagrees with it. Change is challenging when we have been surrounded by weight stigma all our lives and are just now realizing that there is another way. It feels like swimming upstream against the current.

When healers make assumptions based on body size, there is a risk for harm. Nurses take blood pressure multiple times when they cannot believe that a large person could have good numbers. Counselors and psychotherapists offer weight loss advice for complaints of depression. Physical therapists anticipate that a larger person will be too lazy to complete exercises at home. Dieticians routinely offer recommendations for cutting calorie intake. Doctors recommend weight loss without inquiring about possible disordered eating behaviors. Offices are designed without consideration for those who might not fit into a standard chair. Scales may be in waiting rooms or other non-private spaces.

Those who have a diagnosable eating disorder are harmed by this, but so are those with sub-clinical symptoms of disordered eating. Most fat people have spent at least some, perhaps most, of their lives engaging in disordered eating in pursuit of the impossible goal of weight loss, often at the recommendation of their doctors. Eating disorder behaviors include restrictive eating, a preoccupation with weight loss that may interfere with life activities, frequent weighing, self-esteem that is strongly tied to body shape/size, excessive exercise, and feelings of guilt and shame related to eating (National Institute of Mental Health, 2016). These are often the very behaviors that are encouraged in the pursuit of weight loss. When someone has been told to lose weight for health reasons, they engage in these behaviors without even realizing they could be harmful and are often unaware

DOI: 10.4324/9781003057000-2

that what they are doing could be considered problematic. Disordered eating looks like "following the doctor's orders." Disordered eating is the norm. Body dissatisfaction is the norm. The fact that it is common does not mean that it is benign (Mond et al., 2013). Some studies have estimated that as much as 75% of women in America have symptoms of disordered eating (Carolina Public Health, 2008). Weight stigma causes both eating disorders and disordered eating.

I have worked in the eating disorder treatment field for 35 years and I am continually surprised at the lack of awareness of potential harm among medical professionals and lack of concern when it is pointed out. As an example, a couple of years ago a doctor was on a local radio talk show expounding on the apparently limitless benefits of intermittent fasting. When specifically asked, he said that people did not even need to check with their doctors before undertaking it. I contacted him and we had a conversation by email. When I pointed out that his recommendations could be harmful to those with disordered eating, it was clear that such a thing had never crossed his mind. He then said that they should check with their treatment providers, contradicting what he had said on the air. This also ignored the fact that many of those with eating disorders and disordered eating are not in treatment and often do not realize they have a problem. After all, they are only doing what they have been told to do to lose weight.

The weight-loss paradigm that has dominated the medical field is not helping anyone; in fact, it is causing harm (Bacon & Aphramor, 2011). How do we change that? First, we educate ourselves about weight stigma and its effects. Then we need to put that knowledge into practice in the work that we do as well as educational programs in our respective fields.

How do we intentionally create a space for healing that is welcoming and safe to all body sizes? Data and science are necessary to good care, but stories are essential for developing empathy and understanding. Hearing about personal examples of the harm caused by weight stigma in medical care can improve our understanding in a way that facts cannot manage. The following chapters offer a rich mix of science, data, and personal experience.

References

Bacon, L., & Aphramor, L. (2011). Weight science: Evaluating the evidence for a paradigm shift. *Nutrition Journal, 10*(9), 1–13. https://doi.org/10.1186/1475-2891-10-9

Carolina Public Health. (2008). Survey finds disordered eating behaviors among three out of four American women. *Carolina Public Health Magazine.* https://sph.unc.edu/cphm/carolina-public-health-magazine-accelerate-fall-2008/survey-finds-disordered-eating-behaviors-among-three-out-of-four-american-women-fall-2008/

Mond, J., Mitchison, D., Latner, J., Hay, P., Owen, C., & Rodgers, B. (2013). Quality of life impairment associated with body dissatisfaction in a general population sample of women. *BMC Public Health, 13*(920), 1–11. https://doi.org/10.1186/1471-2458-13-920

National Institute of Mental Health. (2016). Eating disorders. https://www.nimh.nih.gov/health/topics/eating-disorders/index.shtml

2 Deadweight

Unpacking fat shame in psychotherapy

Catherine Baker-Pitts

Fat shame—on either side of the therapy couch—is, like deadweight, an excess burden. While the body positivity movement blossoms outside of our consulting rooms, a fat affirmative stance has eluded many psychotherapists who, like the people who come to us seeking emotional refuge, live in a fat phobic culture. This chapter addresses mental health clinicians who regard fatness as a problem to be resolved, a symptom of inner conflict or compulsive eating, and weight loss or thinness as a sign of adaptive adjustment. Associations of fatness with disgust, anxiety, fear, and dread need to be named and analyzed in patients—and confronted in therapists who harbor disdain for what is actually a neutral adjective (Fahs, 2019). Fat bodies are, after all, relative and contingent on changing definitions, contexts, and relationships. In the therapy encounter, the fat body is not the problem but rather it is internalized fat shame—born and cultivated in relationships—that needs unpacking.

The Health Care Rights Law of 2020, intended to guard patients against discrimination on the basis of race, color, national origin, sex, age, and disability in health programs and activities that receive federal funding, does not protect people who are discriminated against on the basis of body size. Even across *therapeutic* settings, body size-based microaggressions, intentional, or unconscious hostile remarks or ideas that are directed at fat people as a group, are rampant and barely acknowledged, much less identified as injurious and unethical (Munro, 2017). Psychologist Breanne Fahs (2019) describes weight bias and the tendency to measure a fat patient's progress by pounds as the most "frankly destructive and grotesquely unreflective" (p. 245) misstep perpetrated by clinicians, who generally pride themselves on offering a contemplative stance, sitting with feelings rather than rushing to action, and eschewing binary thinking in order to hold ambiguity and complexity.

More than 50 years after the 1969 Stonewall riots for gay and transgender liberation, mental health institutes in the United States began issuing formal apologies for the profession's role in pathologizing people of marginalized genders and sexualities. They vowed to interrogate cis, heteronormative, paternalistic theoretical models and prevalent blind spots in practice, ethics, and intellectual discourse. A year later, in 2020, in response to ongoing cultural violence against people of color, these institutes joined the chorus of Black Lives Matter,

DOI: 10.4324/9781003057000-3

acknowledging racial biases within academia and promising to root out systemic racism as it manifests in theoretical whitewashing and racialized encounters in treatment settings (Jones, 2020). Time will tell if any of this is more than what Black therapist Resmaa Menaken (in Tippett, 2020) critically calls the trend of speaking up as "performance art," or public virtue signaling. While training institutes are grappling with past injuries perpetrated in the name of healing, a White European legacy still undergirds much of psychoanalytic theory.

Calls for reckoning with anti-fat bias in our canons, practices, and institutions are woefully absent, with few exceptions (e.g., see Calogero et al., 2019, devoted to ending sizeism). Upending normative psychoanalysis—including shining a skeptical light on the medical model, decentering dominant voices, and attending to intersectional forces (Sheehi, 2020)—will require a fundamental reframing of how we understand fat bodies alongside consumer capitalism, systems of violence, and the politics of love and self-care.

Here I urge psychotherapists to commit ethically to do something about anti-fat bias (see Kinavey & Cool, 2019) within a gender-expansive, anti-racism framework: first, to recognize anti-sizeism in unison with anti-racism practices, as a critical response to the oppressive force of a White, thin, Western beauty standard. It is on the good conscience of practitioners to be skeptical of headlines with alarming assertions about body size, as if to be fat is a crime or a death sentence. It is incumbent on all of us to recognize thinness as a social advantage at the expense of fat people and to interrupt sizeism in ourselves and among colleagues who, for instance, interpret the meaning of the fat body—most predictably as an emotional barrier, or as a container of trauma and neglect—without tending to the cultural degradation and the cumulative trauma of fat hatred. Our critical analysis will be therapeutic only when it accounts for structural inequalities that marginalize people who may have overlapping identities (and who may experience privileges as well) and relates to them as experts in and of their own lives (Nash, 2013).

Shame-based: The misinterpretation of fat bodies

Any of us who studied psychology in graduate school was likely assigned Irvin Yalom as required reading. In his chapter "Fat Lady," Yalom (1989) openly shares his hatred of fat women. He decides to treat a fat patient, Betty, because the "unruly feelings" she elicits represent "the ultimate countertransference challenge"—more challenging than his work with incarcerated people charged with the most heinous crimes, he tells us. Yalom dates his fat hatred to his immigrant youth, when he needed someone lower on the social ladder to mock:

> In the streets, the Blacks attacked me for my Whiteness, and in school, the Whites attacked me for my Jewishness. But there was always fatness, the fat kids, the big asses, the butts of jokes, those last chosen for athletic teams, those unable to run the circle of the athletic track. I needed someone to hate, too. Maybe this is where it began. (p. 88)

Yalom did not expect Betty to perceive his negative feelings, but of course she did. So, too, did the readers who took offense. But Yalom is comforted by the fan mail from clinicians who shared their gratitude for his "courage" in sharing—or unloading—his fat repulsion. As students in training discuss the case of Betty, they might consider the extent to which Yalom's disclosure is in the service of ameliorating his own fat bias or whether his meanderings on the topic are toxic in themselves, exacerbating the persecution of the stigmatized "other."

Curiously, as Fahs (2019) recognizes, psychoanalysts like Yalom who otherwise privilege thoughtful reflection are prone to rush to action when a patient is fat. And when they do *not* rush to address a patient's fat body as a problem worthy of exploration, this is characterized as "collusion" or a "joint dissociation" on the analyst's part rather than as decent respect and open curiosity. This despite the fact that thin, conforming bodies are rarely read as expressing a fragile self-worth or as a symptom of over-compliance with diet culture (Bloom et al., 1994).

In another case in point, psychoanalyst Frank Lachmann (2010) details his work with a patient named Robin, centered on an action-oriented solution to her "weight problem." In an homage to Heinz Kohut's use of "enactments"—the organization of meaning that is implicit, without reflective thought or verbal dialogue—as a road to empathy, Lachmann describes clinical moments in which he listens to and sympathizes with Robin's body shame, including her feelings of abandonment and betrayal by a past lover; he grows concerned, albeit in a patronizing manner, that her weight, which he suspects was the culprit of her romantic failures, cannot be managed by "conscious control or alteration." Unable to sit with the emotional weight of his patient's experience, the therapist determines that "something more" is needed. The enactment, played out by both members of the dyad, is captured by the therapist's suggestion that they should walk together in the park during their allotted session times. He asks Robin to weigh herself weekly and report back to him.

Lachmann describes his intervention as "intuitive" and "empathic," a response to having "felt at a loss as to how to pursue her weight problem given that she would not consider participating in a diet and exercise program." During their (outdoor, walking) sessions, Robin shares that her parents had encouraged her to perform for them. "Of course, she did so," Lachmann (2010) writes, "feeling terrified but never complaining." He professes repeatedly to feel sympathy for Robin's plight, even as he consciously enacts his fat bias in a denigrating manner during their sessions together.

As I read these clinical vignettes, my thoughts are guided by the ideas of feminist psychoanalytic pioneers like Clara Thompson (1938, 1943, 1945), who thought a lot about the internalization of pernicious forces in the culture. She challenged Freud's assertions about the inferiority complex, which he tied directly to a female's biology, and developed her clinical understanding with attunement to cultural conditions—restrictions on women's freedom and intellectual pursuits, expectations of matrimony and motherhood, anxieties about a girl's developing body, for instance—that bred under-privilege.

In 1940, Thompson described a psychological maneuver called "identification with the enemy and loss of the sense of self," whereby children take on the attitudes and behaviors of people whom they love and admire. Motivated primarily by fear, the child joins with hostile forces, entwining their identity and identifications with others. Growing up, the child adopts the mentality of the "powerful other" for protective reasons, but in this move they also lose the ability to assess the minds and motives of others; to avoid disapproval, they latch on tightly, an unconscious defense strategy of identifying out of fear.

For people of whom compliance was expected in early life, this dynamic likely plays out with the therapist as uncritical identification, again to preserve the attachment. When a person is not encouraged to have their own mind, to think for themselves, or to disagree with authorities, but is instead expected to surrender their own thoughts and join with the other, the capacity for emboldened action and self-determination is lost. In the co-created enactment Lachmann and Robin engage in, the therapist does not appreciate his patient's fear of speaking up, of disappointing the authority, of complaining about being misunderstood. "I am sure my parents would have responded," Robin says at one point, "but I thought I just had to do it"—a revelation met with silence. On top of this, as psychotherapist Linda Arbus (personal conversation, August 23, 2020) speculates based on her own experience, Robin likely suffered from a lack of entitlement to voice resistance due to the cumulative toll of body shame and fat stigma the enemy internalized over many years.

In yet another shame-based intervention, psychoanalyst Caryn Sherman-Meyer (2015) describes her work as a fat therapist who "through her own integration of previously dissociated fat hatred" addresses the shame and guilt "of being fat and hating fat." Her fat loathing, she surmises, led to "attacks on fat linking," which she describes as an avoidance of fatness—its meaning and associations—in the therapy relationship. She revisits how she and one patient, Liv, collude in not talking about their "shared heaviness," as though Liv's non-issue with her body signals self-neglect. Like so many others, Sherman-Meyer (2015) regards fatness as a problem—a psychological defense, such as a protection or deterrent against intimacy—that is only resolved when the fat vanishes.

As Saguy (2012) contends, responses to fat have everything to do with how it is contextualized or schematically perceived—that is, "framed." Fat is framed in our society, foremost, as a serious problem, whether as a medical disease, a public health crisis, or as an indicator of individual immorality and weakness. In truth, people of all sizes avoid not only psychotherapists, but also medical doctors, gyms, social gatherings, professional opportunities, and recreation parks due to fears of encountering the "blame frame," whereby body weight is attributed to personal failure and lack of will, blamed for all ailments for which weight loss is prescribed as the best solution (Saguy, 2012). So, it is of little surprise that Liv found comfort and hoped for reparative healing in her attachment to a fat therapist. During the treatment, as Sherman-Meyer (2015) actively loses weight, Liv apparently experiences feelings of loss connected to the disappearance of the other fat body in the room. The thinning therapist interprets her reaction as mounting anger and jealousy—which, Sherman-Meyer suggests, ushers in a period of what she refers to as differentiation.

In this case, Sherman-Meyer (2015) imposes her own agenda on the patient, who perceives the conflict her therapist is facing: "I really think that my staying fat is an emotional thing for you," Liv intuits. When Liv claims that she is not so bothered by her fat body, Sherman-Meyer (2015) is incredulous, and concludes that she has merely dissociated her fat hatred. Sherman-Meyer's baggage of biases or what she calls her "fat-hating internal world" perpetuates the cultural phobia of fat in her relationship with Liv, which begs a question: how can patients undo a traumatically preoccupied body image if a psychotherapist is fixated on body size? Convinced that weight loss signals superior health, the therapist does not make room for an alternative narrative in which a fat person is not fat-hating, sabotaging, or "resistant."

In a twist of care, Liv offers to her therapist the body acceptance that the patient herself craves; Liv is more evolved in this regard than many. In response to a large-bodied therapist, the transference of distrust, as defensive as it clearly is, often goes unquestioned. In finding a therapist for her daughter, a patient I work with named Ellen was reluctant to accept a referral to a therapist who seemed best suited to her daughter's needs because of the therapist's body size. The therapist's fatness, Ellen presumed, signaled something about her self-care practices and by extension, her ability to care for the daughter. The mother, Ellen, smokes heavily, bikes recklessly all over Manhattan, barely sleeps because of anxiety, and seeps into reckless mood swings, and yet she leaps to rash judgments of a fat therapist, making her the unknowing container of Ellen's own feared and hated parts. The crux of Ellen's therapy centers on understanding how her critical judgments of others create for her a persecutory environment in which vigilance is required and nobody is safe.

Without an anti-racist, body-affirmative stance, all of us—fat, thin, of any size—are at risk of dwelling in body shame and spreading weight-based biases, regardless of how many hours we have spent analyzing our minds. For some people—perhaps like Sherman-Meyer, and certainly for 50-year-old Sarah Miller, who penned "Fat Me, Skinny Me, and the Diet Industrial Complex" for *The New York Times* (March 1, 2020)—fat shame is deeply entrenched and intractable, so much so in Miller's case that she feels it is simply unfeasible to undo. In the piece, she acknowledges that fat-affirming voices from the cultural surround cannot soften the critique within when a body is saturated by a lifetime of size-based humiliation. "Even if I don't shame others," Miller laments, "I can't stop fat shaming myself."

I have been on the receiving end of a therapist's hang-ups about fat. Roughly 30 years ago, when I was a teenager, I realized just how influential, loaded, and deleterious a therapeutic intervention can be. I had been directed to a therapist to talk about my feelings in the days after my family learned that I had been sexually assaulted months earlier. I recall my disappointment that the therapist's body was so lean and sinewy, without any soft spots. After making little headway in opening me up, the hard-bodied therapist directed her intervention to the surface level: she wondered if I might take up jogging and consider ingesting fewer bagels. If I could control my appetite and my body, she suggested, I might gain a feeling of body ownership.

As it turned out, this therapist-endorsed body preoccupation did distract me from feeling my vulnerability and my dread about my maturing body, but it also did me a great disservice in the long term, as I lost precious years to bizarre symptoms that interfered with my curiosity, my intellectual interests, my attunement to my sexuality, and more. What helped me eventually develop these parts of myself were "gender outlaws" intent on abolishing prescriptive gender assignments and social movements working against sizeism—which gave me the courage to question the diet apparatus's demands for body conformity, derision of dissent, and diminishing of largesse in people who have much to gain by way of social change.

Finding validation and inspiration in social protests is not specific to me. Jeannine Gailey's (2012) interviews with women about their dating and sexual experiences indicate that fat pride and engagement with the size acceptance movement helps to ameliorate body shame. The more I recognized fat hatred as being entwined with gender, race, and class oppression, the greater my investment grew in confronting body bashing—whether in the form of fat talk, objectification, or slut shaming—of myself or others. If fighting fat phobia cured me of an adolescent eating problem, it also shaped me as a therapist. I grew to understand that the cultural denigration of fat is a form of social control that impedes mental health and keep all bodies in check.

Thin fragility

Buttressed by an ideology referred to as both benevolent sizeism (Chrisler & Barney, 2017) and healthism, which serves to rationalize weight bias and compulsory weight loss interventions, thin supremacy—and its cousin, thin fragility—shows up in the form of superiority, defensiveness, and entitlement. It is an aggressive response to humanizing perspectives of fat people that conceals hostility towards fatness with condescension. Both White supremacy and thin supremacy, rooted in an unsavory history of colonialism, work in the service of defending the status quo. Pseudo-scientific assertions of biologically based differences and hierarchies, particularly in reference to racialized bodies, have long been used to justify hatred in the guise of knowledge (Woods, 2020).

Fatness is referred to in media, public health, and medical literature as a "disease" that threatens health care systems and requires behavioral change at the level of the individual, family, and community (Trainer et al., 2015). In public discourse, fat bodies are marked as marginal and therefore deserving of suspicion and public interrogation, in need of personal vigilance, especially non-White fat bodies. For example, while nations closed their borders to contain the spread of the coronavirus, Britain's prime minister sounded the alarm on the medicalized "obesity epidemic," publicly haranguing his own and others' midsections.[1]

Social monitoring focused on "health" quickly morphed into an issue of entitlement to space, accentuating structural problems and scapegoating fat bodies—and Black bodies too. Strings (2020) names the twin pandemics of racism and fat stigma as being inextricably entwined. Linking the hatred of fatness in our culture to the fear of Black bodies, Strings (2020) explicates the historical racialized, gendered, social hierarchies that have degraded Black (fat) women and elevated White (thin) women, perpetuating fat aversion and thin preoccupation, throughout history. Farrell (2011) likewise explores fatness as a crucial marker in an economic hierarchy that deems thin bodies as civilized while it links fat bodies to adjectives reserved for those who constitute the dregs of society: primitive, degenerate, dependent, and uncivilized.

Kendi (2019) describes "space racism" as a powerful collection of racist policies that lead to resource inequity, substantiated by racist ideas about racialized spaces. In parallel, space sizeism is the product of inhospitable environments and weight-based policies that impinge on fat people's access and mobility. A patient I work with, Gemma, described an argument centered on space sizeism with her boyfriend, who was insisting that fat people should pay more to secure space on a flight. Flexing his normative-bodied privilege, his fat revulsion surfaced as he described the claustrophobia of bodies touching. He could not conceive that spaces ought to be made to accommodate everyone. This topic is not distant or hypothetical to Gemma; her ability to live soundly in her body depends on a benign space for her body to be free of scrutiny.

So long as thinness is upheld as superior to fatness, or weight loss is conflated with health, or the scientific method is touted to bolster or justify harassing fat patients, therapists will be practicing within an assimilationist framework, perpetuating space sizeism. About White supremacy, Menaken (in Tippett, 2020) states, racist culture has "tenderized physical systems to the point where COVID-19 set up shop because our bodies were already murdered." Menaken insists, Black bodies are weathered by the social trauma of racism. Fat bodies, too, are weathered by social trauma—fattism is encountered on airline travel and in doctor's offices, movie theatres, restaurants, therapy offices, and on and on.

When fat people are referred to as "obese," for instance, the commentary is distant and reductive, as it generalizes about bodies without knowledge of how psychological and sociocultural stressors, such as social disapproval (Bruno, 2017), for any given person, map onto biology. Just as racial disparities in health have to do with societal ills, a growing body of research shows that encounters with weight bias and stigma are health offenses that adversely affect stress levels, economic status, and longevity (Puhl et al., 2020).

Thinness, not unlike Whiteness, still operates as an idealized standard by which other body types are judged. Different from race, body size is perceived as malleable, a non-fixed status; social mobility is offered through the portal of dieting. Kendi (2019) refers to Black people who have "made it" by the standards of dominant culture as "the exceptionals" and insists, "Assimilationist ideas are racist ideas" (January 29, 2019, Twitter). Fat people are uniformly sold weight loss interventions with the promise of moving out of a stigmatized group (Throsby, 2008) in a sort of assimilationist logic. Fat people who, like Oprah Winfrey, lose weight "successfully" are indeed exceptional—and the assimilationist ideas (e.g., weight watchers) they push on others about dieting are weightist ideas. Rather than supporting weight loss, psychotherapists might instead ask, what else is lost for the person who aspires to shed a marginalized identity? As L. Arbus (personal communication, August 23, 2020) conveys, praise and validation based on changing one's body are conditional and thus undermine the experience of being seen and truly accepted in one's own right, unaltered. Furthermore, even people for whom weight loss is felt as an exceptional achievement endure the dread—the looming sword of Damocles—of regaining weight.

Living in a Black body: "A low-level dread"

The conflation of fatness with disease is not only out there in public opinion; it also burrows as a critical voice within. Fifty-two-year-old Cressida[2], a Black woman with a solid, statuesque frame, dreads visiting her cardiologist; she has other concerns to address yet she is filled with shame in anticipation of his scolding grimace about her weight.

Cressida sought psychotherapy as a place to let down her guard. She desired self-awareness, preferably coupled with weight loss. Early in our work, I gently suggested that my hope was to help her grow, not shrink; to gain a deeper understanding of her inner and interpersonal worlds; and to locate the source of her internalized body inferiority. I hoped we would get there with curiosity and compassion.

Now, in the midst of the COVID-19 quarantine, Cressida flagellates herself for seeking comfort from a nightly bowl of ice cream, as though hers is not a perfectly human—and harmless—desire, while anti-racism demonstrations erupt just outside her door in Harlem. Rather than joining the protesters, she stays tucked mostly inside her home, embroiled in battles with her teenage child, who is on the autism spectrum and who is growing tall and broad like herself. Their conflict centers on cookies and online consumption, both of which she tries to manage without success. I press Cressida about the predictable outcome of these power struggles with her son and the isolation and loneliness they each endure. Eventually we arrive at a source of her body loathing, as she describes her "low-level dread" about her child's vulnerability to racial profiling and violence, an anxiety that grows in proportion to his body size. The surveillance she feels on behalf of her son, and the ways that she monitors him, are pointedly about his survival.

Cressida also worries about her 10-year-old daughter's developing body, which reminds Cressida of her own school-age experiences of being treated as "different" and being marginalized in her mostly White classrooms. As a nurturing parent, she knows not to focus on her child's appearance; she emphasizes what her daughter's body can do (fitness!) instead. Even these coded messages, I fear, betray Cressida's unsettled relationship with her own and, by extension, her daughter's body. At moments, I recognize my own feelings of futility in helping Cressida to reframe and soften her fat associations; my fervent anti-diet stance refuses to see Cressida's or her children's appetites and bodies as problems to be contained.

Jennifer Nash (2013) situates the modern-day work of self-care by Black women as a revolutionary act; if not culturally bred into Black females, self-love is learned as part of a political struggle. And this is where Cressida is most vulnerable, but racial difference looms large between us. As Cressida speaks openly and unapologetically about her body hatred with me, I wonder if weight complaints might be the democratic equalizer between us; after all, fat phobia is one of the last socially acceptable forms of prejudice across racial groups in the United States. Cressida describes her feelings of body inferiority and her envy of people for whom, she says, "life just works out, a category to which she suspects I belong.

She refers only obliquely to race, and yet Cressida opted for a White therapist. I wonder if our racial difference allows her to accentuate her Blackness, while exploring her conflictual racial identifications. She tells me about the profound disappointment she felt when she was accepted at an Ivy League university, a story she shares again and again, like a relational trauma to be repeated and remembered. Despite her conviction that it was the best school for her, she was forbidden to attend the elite institution by her father, himself an academic at a historically Black college, as if to do so would be a betrayal of her Black allegiance.

Before the influence and transparency of the analyst's subjectivity was appreciated, Thompson (1938, 1943, 1945) was clear that the attitudes of the analyst have a bearing on a patient's experience of treatment. Cressida perceives my biases in our interactions and in my aesthetic choices, gestures, and thoughts. A key conflict between us centers on my distrust of traditional institutions, like Boy Scouts of America where she sends her son, and my refusal to endorse her weight-loss strategies. As she describes what feels to her like the mocking presence of her Peloton bike, a pricey piece of equipment that occupies space in her home, I wonder if Cressida has internalized the classist view that women whose bodies do not conform to White elite norms can be empowered to make what Anna Kirkland (2010) calls "virtuous personal consumer choices," given the opportunity. Perhaps in response to feeling at a loss in finding help from me in her desire to conform to thin beauty norms, without any mention, she traveled to attend a week-long weight-focused retreat, led by a body guru in another state, where she was the sole Black participant. I wonder if she did not tell me for fear that I, like her father, would criticize her "uppity" choices. She notices when I grow impatient with her submission to her Peloton and her longing for approval from status culture. Desperate to rattle her, I share that I feel angry on her behalf—at her weight preoccupied husband, at her cardiologist, at her size-obsessed friends who taunt her with their diets. And she lets me know what she thinks in the abstract of "White progressives," those people who "say all the right things but don't adequately pay the people who take care of their kids."

Occasionally, Cressida imagines "just giving up" on her arts career or on dieting pursuits—the ultimate failure—in her mind. Thompson writes, "… even when a woman has become consciously convinced of her value she still has to contend with the unconscious effects of training, discrimination against her, and traumatic experiences which keep alive the attitude of inferiority" (1942, p. 233). In my utopian view, I long for Cressida to let go of diminishing messages that inhibit her as she defends against getting angry at the source of racism and sizeism—a whole cultural setup that disadvantages her.

Our work together culminates in an enactment in which Cressida sees my liberal strivings, like my push against fattism, as vanity projects, out of touch with her realities. She lets me know that she distrusts my need for her to resist to cultural norms. In our initial meetings, I did misinterpret Cressida, perhaps out of my desire for her sensibility to match what I, in a racialized stereotype, observed as an unconventional image. Her glistening makeup-free skin and her natural African American hair were not, as I imagined, countercultural. Her at-home work-out equipment does, in fact, signal a wish to be aligned with bourgeois values. None of that eases the blows of racism, sizeism, and sexism she has been dealt at every turn in the image-obsessed industry in which she works. When I ask if I am included in her dig about "White progressives," she shrugs and suggests, imperceptibly, "I don't know?" as if asking if I live by the ideals of body acceptance that I promote. My ideas are far removed from her lived experience.

My wish for Cressida to become more defiant against diet mandates and her response of doubling down on the pursuit of the thin ideal, I come to appreciate, highlights a turn toward difference, rather than sameness, between us. In a very real sense, Cressida accurately perceives my privilege: I, a White person, can fight for racial justice, body size acceptance, and gender creativity from a non-Black, non-fat, non-trans, and non-marginalized position. My push for size diversity is suspicious, as I benefit from and embody the power structures that I am critiquing, a shame I must manage. I cannot escape my proximity to systems that oppress, just as Cressida inhabits a body that is the site of societal projections that do not recognize her.

The visibility of Cressida's body has been a liability, I learn more and more; she does not wish to stick out, either with radical ideas or with an exceptional appearance. She devotes abundant attention to helping her child who is on the spectrum adapt to mainstream culture; she supports him to familiarize himself with and imitate, literally, the presentation of his neurotypical peers. She does not want to—nor should she have to—deal with the costs of non-conformity. In her Black body, she is in harm's way by state-sanctioned violence and prevalent racism in ways that I am not. In fact, her ability to express her criticism of me directly—even in her refusal to champion the cause of size acceptance—marks a therapeutic gain. It is at least a step toward opening up hostilities, externalizing her anger, and, I hope, affirming her own mind.

In Thompson's clinical practice, young women described the harsh restrictions they encountered as they matured into womanhood, including "feelings of body shame, loss of freedom, loss of equality with boys, and loss of the right to be aggressive" (1942, p. 335). Today, a thinness complex may signal the tremendous burden of race, class, gender, and body-size oppression. Where Thompson (1950) focused her inquiry on what "being a woman" meant to her patient at a time when penis envy had little to do with an organ and everything to do with social opportunities that favored men, my clinical mind veers to what thinness means—and more specifically the ways that being a woman, a Black woman, map onto being a fat woman for Cressida. As I recognize our different subjectivities, I can attend to the ways that, for Cressida, her body can feel to her like a disappointment and an obstacle, something to be gotten rid of. With permission not to change, I feel relieved to hear Cressida's plea for room to voice her outsized feelings. Now I listen for what the idealized body confers, at least in fantasy: a certain freedom from judgment, a valuing of oneself, self-contentment, and social privilege that feels inaccessible to her, despite her affluence and education. Thompson realized even in 1950, "that the acceptance of one's body and all its functions is a basic need in the establishment of self-respect and self-esteem" (p. 253).

Capsized: Navigating a way out of fat shame

In order to guide liberatory change in ourselves and our institutions, serious introspection, humble curiosity, and a spirited effort to take back the shame that has been disowned and projected onto fat people will be needed. Therapists who assert a "neutral," size-free perspective, but offer little in the way of fat affirmation, cannot provide the breakwater needed when a person is saturated by fat shame; just as "not being a racist" is different than anti-racism (Kendi, 2019), a claim of weight neutrality does not affirm for fat people either their bodies or the validity of their suffering in a fat shaming culture. The cultural logics of body affirmative care are tied to anti-racism; there is no in-between in the struggle for body size equity. Either a therapist is reproducing the problem by harboring an individualistic blame frame (Saguy, 2012) or they are actively committed to undoing weight bias, predicated on a system of attitudes and policies that discriminate against and disadvantage people of size, whether the bias shows up explicitly or implicitly, consciously or unconsciously. Nobody, including me, is exempt from the emotional labor and inconvenience required of us to interrupt the problematic ways we have been conditioned in a size phobic, racist environment.

I actively challenged Cressida's defenses against self-acceptance, for example, but a key turning point in our work came when I accepted that my intervention, intellectualized as it is, might underestimate the psychological pull and currency of at least striving to lose weight for some people (see Penney & Kirk, 2015). I pivoted to accept Cressida's need for the thin fantasy as entwined with our difference, while she rejected my anti-dieting stance. Without this acknowledgment, herein lies what Thompson (1938, 1943, 1945) would call my "weak spots"—my blindness to my own normative bodied, raced privilege. By disavowing my guilt and over-identifying with the "outsider," my anti-racist, anti-sizeist worldview misses Cressida. I shifted within myself to recognize that Cressida is already dealing with "trouble" in her life, including the care of a child who faces multiple perils at the intersection of ableism, racism, and sizeism. She should not take on my wish for her to be the poster child of a striving, large, self-contented Black woman.

In a virtual session, Cressida downplayed the news of what is a massive career achievement, and then proceeded to spend the bulk of our time belittling her body.

I try to sink into her feeling that her body is a burden, while calling attention to the ways that she preemptively cuts herself down in response to feeling big and proud.

"Do you notice that you went right to attacking your body just when your accomplishment was announced, when your hard work—your hunger for this project—became visible?"

She confided, "With anything good, something always levels me."

"Why dream of the Ivy Tower if you can't actually go?" I asked. Cressida recollected her gleeful anticipation, years before, – when her first child picked up a second language easily and her pride when he showed signs of advanced reading and writing—and the crushing blow of learning that his precociousness actually set him apart from his mainstream neurotypical peers. To dream, she told me, is risky.

Now, back to that unhelpful therapist of mine, who did not enable me to trust and love my developing adolescent body. Instead of helping me to own my anger at the boys who had assaulted me or at the institution that had doubled down on my shame by shrouding the assault in secrecy and silence for months, this therapist imparted to me self-scrutiny and self-restraint. She taught me how to run from my feelings and to hide my curves. While I was stuck on a concrete measure of fat in terms of inches and garment sizes, I really needed help unpacking the *feeling* of fat, which had everything to do with my self-blame and shame about being too outgoing and trusting, and nothing at all to do with my body. What if, instead of being prescribed activities to control my body, I had been able to challenge the therapist's intervention, her worldview that bodies ought to be controlled? What if I had questioned the premise that changing my body would offer me a modicum of safety?

In a just world, therapists would own responsibility, address their own anti-fat bias and make reparations to patients who have been harmed by fat hatred. It is on us to be mindful and to strive to grow bigger in the fight to unlearn racism and sizeism. To the extent that fat phobia represents a health crisis, we need to turn our attention to the ways in which discrimination and stigma impact health and status in society (Brownell et al., 2005). We need to stop forcing people to mold themselves into shapes that make others comfortable; being fat, after all, is a fundamental right (Calogero et al., 2019).

In *Hunger*, Roxane Gay (2017) takes to task the societal disciplining of what she calls her "unruly body." In a subsequent narrative, she shares that she felt compelled to change her body by drastic means because of the agony of fat hatred when cultural progress is slow-going. Recently, Cressida pointed me this article written by Gay, after weight-loss surgery, in which the author claims, "As my body contracted, my world expanded." While Cressida focuses on the potential to fit in, to hide the torment of living in a body that is unwelcome in a racist, size-unfriendly world, I tune into Gay's desire to accept herself, to embrace her hungers, however big and messy. Gay addresses these dueling needs while marveling at how internalized fat shame has limited her. If she had not been apologetic in her fat body, might she have savored a Parisian loaf or enjoyed a Venetian gelato sooner, she wonders?

As COVID-19 continues to limit the labor of social engagements, Cressida reports feeling less burdened by her body. To clarify, I ask if her own view in the mirror troubles her less, or if she feels some respite out of public view, without scrutiny focused on her body. Cressida's face on Zoom brightens as she shares that, after collectively enduring a quarantine, "it's just a relief that everyone is looking a little schlubby." In place of humiliation, she notices, she feels permission; hopeful, I ask if she might be able to carry the freedom she feels in this moment from the gaze into the world. During a time that has brought to the fore a global reckoning with White supremacy and the enticing potential for social change, might Cressida have room for self-love, "regardless," described by Alice Walker as a "political event" that is "absolutely essential, that it persists in spite of everything else" (Nash, 2013, p. 10)? Cressida's face relaxes and as she looks out her window, she exhales.

Regardless of the trouble any of us might feel in our bodies and in our culture, isn't a life of self-love and pleasure—with texture and sweetness, as Gay eventually discovered—a worthy therapeutic aim? And if in a process of discovering anti-capitalist sources of self-value we become more whole, kind, and less shame-filled, might we extend to the public sphere a politics of care and affirmation? Imagine the potential for deep transformation if we could make room for, as Nash (2016, p. 11) envisions, "the vibrancy and complexity of difference." In my work with Cressida, I have been humbled by the shame that is generated—and softened—in relationship. A full embrace of Cressida, just as she is, marks a new day for both of us.

Special thanks

I am indebted to Mikaela Luttrell-Rowland and Linda Arbus for valuable theoretical clarity and broad-minded feedback on this chapter—and all things social justice.

Notes

1 Tucked within journalistic articles shouting the risks of obesity are offhand remarks about the editorial nature of their bold claims and cautionary tales—"the research is preliminary and not peer reviewed, but it buttresses anecdotal reports. .," admits Boris Johnson's "New Tactic Against the Virus: Urge Britons to Lose Weight," published in *The New York Times*.
2 Name changed to protect anonymity.

References

Bloom, C., Gitter, A., Gutwill, S., Kogel, L., & Zaphiropoulos, L. (1994). *Eating problems: A feminist psychoanalytic treatment model*. Basic Books.
Brownell, K., Puhl, R., Schwartz, M., & Rudd, L. (Eds.). (2005). *Weight bias: Nature, consequences, and remedies*. Guildford Publications.
Bruno, B. A. (2017). Health at Every Size and me. *Fat Studies*, 6(1), 54–66. https://doi.org/10.1080/21604851.2016.1218741

Calogero, R., Tylka, T., Mensinger, J., Meadows, A., & Daníelsdóttir, S. (2019). Recognizing the fundamental right to be fat: A weight-inclusive approach to size acceptance and healing from sizeism. *Women & Therapy*, 42(1–2), 22–44. https://doi.org/10.1080/02703149.2018.1524067

Chrisler, J., & Barney, A. (2017). Sizeism is a health hazard. *Fat Studies*, 6, 38–53. https://doi.org/10.1080/21604851.2016.1213066

Fahs, B. (2019). Fat and furious: Interrogating fat phobia and nurturing resistance in medical framings of fat bodies. *Women's Reproductive Health*, 6(4), 245–251. https://doi.org/10.1080/23293691.2019.1653577

Farrell, A. E. (2011). *Fat shame: Stigma and the fat body in American culture*. New York University Press.

Gailey, J. A. (2012). Fat shame to fat pride: Fat women's sexual and dating experiences. *Fat Studies*, 1(1), 114–127. https://doi.org/10.1080/21604851.2012.631113

Gay, R. (2017). *Hunger: A memoir of (my) body*. Harper Collins.

Jones, A. L. (2020). A Black woman as an American analyst: Some observations from one woman's life over four decades. *Studies in Gender and Sexuality*, 21(2), 77–84. https://doi.org/10.1080/15240657.2020.1760013

Kendi, I. X. (2019). *How to be an anti-racist*. Random House.

Kirkland, A. (2010). The environmental account for obesity: A case for feminist skepticism. *Signs: Journal of Women in Culture and Society*, 36(2), 1–23.

Kinavey, H., & Cool, C. (2019). The broken lens: How anti-fat bias in psychotherapy is harming our clients and what to do about it. *Women & Therapy*, 42(1–2), 116–130. https://doi.org/10.1080/02703149.2018.1524070

Lachmann, F. M. (2010). Going home. *International Journal of Psychoanalytic Self Psychology*, 5(2), 144–159.

Miller, S. (March 1, 2020). Fat-me, skinny-me, and the diet-industrial complex. *New York Times*, ST, p. 1.

Munro, L. (2017). Everyday indignities: Using the microaggressions framework to understand weight stigma. *The Journal of Law, Medicine & Ethics*, 45(4), 502–509. https://doi.org/10.1177%2F1073110517750584

Nash, J. C. (2013). Practicing love: Black feminism, love-politics, and post-intersectionality. *Meridians*, 11(2), 1–24. https://doi.org/10.2979/meridians.11.2.1

Nash, J. C. (2016). Feminist originalism: Intersectionality and the politics of reading. *Feminist Theory*, 17(1), 3–20. https://doi.org/10.1177%2F1464700115620864

Penney, T. L., & Kirk, S. F. (2015). The Health at Every Size paradigm and obesity: Missing empirical evidence may help push the reframing obesity debate forward. *American Journal of Public Health*, 105(5), e38–e42. https://doi.org/10.2105/AJPH.2015.302552

Puhl, R. M., Himmelstein, M. S., & Pearl, R. I. (2020). Weight stigma as a psychosocial contributor to obesity. *American Psychologist*, 75(2), 274–289. https://doi.org/10.1037/amp0000538

Saguy, A. (2012). *What's wrong with fat?* Oxford University Press.

Sheehi, L. (2020). Talking back introduction to special edition: Black, Indigenous, women of color talk back: Decentering normative psychoanalysis. *Studies in Gender & Sexuality*, 21(2), 73–76. https://doi.org/10.1080/15240657.2020.1760012

Sherman-Meyer, C. (2015). What's fat got to do with it? On different kinds of losses and gains in the analytic relationship. *Psychoanalytic Inquiry*, 35(3), 271–280. https://doi.org/10.1080/07351690.2015.1012461

Strings, S. (2020). *Fearing the Black body: The racial origins of fat phobia*. New York University Press.

Thompson, C. (1938). Notes on the psychoanalytic significance of the choice of the analyst. *Psychiatry, 1*(2), 205–216.

Thompson, C. (1940). Identification with the enemy and loss of the sense of self. *Psychoanalytic Quarterly, 9*(1), 37–50.

Thompson, C. (1942). Cultural pressures in the psychology of women. *Psychiatry, 5*(3), 331–339.

Thompson, C. (1943) "Penis envy" in women. *Psychiatry, 6*(2), 123–125.

Thompson, C. (1945). Transference as a therapeutic instrument. *Psychiatry, 8*(3), 273–278.

Thompson, C. (1950). Some effects of the derogatory attitude toward female sexuality. *Psychiatry: Journal for the Study of Interpersonal Processes, 13*(3), 349–354. https://doi.org/10.1080/00332747.1950.11022785

Tippett, K. (Host). (2020, July 9). Robin DiAngelo and Resmaa Menaken: In conversation [Audio podcast episode]. In *On being*. WNYC Studios. https://onbeing.org/programs/robin-diangelo-and-resmaa-menakem-in-conversation/

Throsby, K. (2008). Happy re-birthday: Weight loss surgery and the "new me." *Body & Society, 4*(1), 117–133. https://doi.org/10.1177%2F1357034X07087534

Trainer, S., Brewis, A., Hruschka, D., & Williams, D. (2015). Translating obesity: Navigating the front lines of the "war on fat." *American Journal of Human Biology, 27*(1), 61–68. https://doi.org/10.1002/ajhb.22623

Woods, A. (2020). The work before us: Whiteness and the psychoanalytic institute. *Psychoanalysis, Culture & Society, 25*(2), 230–249. https://doi.org/10.1057/s41282-019-00155-3

Yalom, I. (1989). *Love's executioner and other tales of psychotherapy*. Perseus Books.

3 Medical equipment

The manifestation of anti-fat bias in medicine

Fady Shanouda

I am scared to get sick. I am not frightened of the consequences of illness—pain, suffering, discomfort, even death. These are inescapable truths. No, I am afraid of being denied the most basic care because I am fat. This fear started when, in an offhand comment, my general practitioner conveyed how difficult it might be for me to get a magnetic resonance imaging (MRI) scan given my size. The same doctor has tried to weigh me by balancing each leg on a different scale and has waved off testing my blood pressure because the cuffs in her office were too small. Medical equipment embodies the anti-fat bias inherent in the medical community (Wann, 2009). Scales, blood pressure cuffs, examination gowns, pelvic examination instruments, MRI and CT scanners, rollators, wheelchairs, hospital beds, even chairs (in waiting rooms and doctors' offices) inform fat patients of their unacceptability as (fat) people. These findings are well documented in the literature (Amy et al., 2006; Diconsiglio, 2006; Kaminsky & Gadaleta, 2002; Merrill & Grassley, 2008; Phelan et al., 2015; Pryor, 2002). However, often absent in these studies are answers to the questions: How did we get here? How did medical equipment become exclusionary?

Many will respond to these questions by pointing to ideas like universal standards or sizes, the notion of the average person, and some might even reference Leonardo da Vinci's drawing of the Vitruvian Man. Others might argue that these are business decisions; that corporations create products to meet or fit the greatest demand. All these responses are valid, albeit misleading. To answer these questions, we have to contend with the social and cultural implications of the eugenics project.

In this chapter, I describe the connections between the eugenics project, the rise and use of statistics, and the impact these had on design principles. I demonstrate how these influenced the development and construction of everyday objects—including medical equipment and testing practices. It is crucial to understand that although I am writing about concepts (statistics, standards, and averages), we often associate with fact or truth—these are, in the end, political ideas that were created, developed, (mis)interpreted, and employed for specific, and at times deadly, purposes. There is a politics behind the construction of the average—the norm, and the ab-normal. The legacy of this politics is what some of us must contend with every time we visit a doctor or try to access health services.

DOI: 10.4324/9781003057000-4

Statistics, eugenics, and design

It might be best to start with Adolphe Quetelet. A Belgian mathematician, among other things, Quetelet is best remembered for his contributions to statistics, and precisely, for his application of comparative statistics to social conditions and moral issues (Eknoyan, 2007). Inspired by work that astronomers used to locate a star—by plotting all the sightings and then averaging the errors—Quetelet applied this idea to human characteristics—at first, height and weight. Davis (2006) argues, however, that Quetelet went a step further when he averaged human data and subsequently developed the concept of the average man. In doing so, Davis (2006) contends that Quetelet created an ideal body—one that was ostensibly in the middle and allowed for no extremes or diversions one way or the other. His approach, referred to as the Quetelet index, was incorporated by many thinkers and academics, including one of his contemporaries—Sir Francis Galton.

Galton, Charles Darwin's cousin, in addition to coining the term "eugenics"—meaning "good-birth" in Greek—also made significant and long-lasting changes to statistics. Davis (2006) tells us that Galton was less interested in charting human variation using Quetelet's index, and instead wanted to ensure that preferred traits, such as being tall and of high intelligence, would be classified as part of the norm—and not as outliers or extremes (as they would on a bell-curve). If Galton applied Quetelet's index without any changes, traits that he defined as preferred would ultimately fall outside the norm. For example, height; rather than having both extremes of height (tall and short) be equally divergent from the norm, Galton instead interpreted statistical curves as ranked quartiles or levels, such that the "extreme positive trait" (being tall, in this example) ranked the highest (Davis, 2006). He referred to these changes when arranged in a chart as an "ogive." These revisions manipulated some characteristics as positive (tallness) and some as deviant and unwanted (shortness) and consequently created the norm as an unattainable standard.

In creating the norm, Davis (2006) argues that Galton also produced the binary elements of disabled and abject—what we might refer to as the non-normative body. Once populations were divided into the norm and the non-norm, and the standard and non-standard, the next step was "for the state to attempt to norm the non-standard" (Davis, 2006, p. 6). Another term to describe these normalizing attempts is eugenics. Eugenics has two distinct branches—positive and negative eugenics. Negative eugenics refers to the mass institutionalization, sterilization, and eradication of certain individuals depending on race, disability, sexuality, and religion. While the Holocaust is the most explicit and deadly example of negative eugenics, there are many contemporary examples of negative eugenics around the world, including the crisis at the southern U.S. border where children are being held in cages or the rise of "re-education camps" in northern China for the minority Muslim population, the Uighurs. Positive eugenics refers to efforts focused on the promotion of "good stock or seed." Laws against interracial marriage (miscegenation laws), caste systems that prevent marriage across class levels, and contemporary efforts at designer babies or genetically reengineered offspring all stem from positive eugenic efforts in the late early and mid-19th century. To summarize, the eugenics project sought to improve the human race by eliminating or preventing the spread of deviant hereditary traits (however those are defined) and through the promotion of both "proper" marriages and healthy offspring (Cogdell, 2010; Davis, 2006; Garland-Thomson, 1997). To think of eugenics as anything less than international in scope, supported by academics, governments, social and cultural institutions, is to underestimate its historical significance and legacy of the movement (Mitchell & Snyder, 2003).

The Quetelet index is now more commonly known as the body mass index (BMI) and has been used incorrectly to measure one's health since 1972, following a study by Ancel Keys (Eknoyan, 2007). One can speak at length about the BMI and its harmful effects; however, others have done this more fully, pointing to the test's mathematical inaccuracies (why square height?) as well as preference toward Eurocentric bodies. It is not lost on me, that the same index manipulated to produce the intended pseudo-science that grounds the project of eugenics is still used by doctors today to measure (and help erase) fat people's bodies. The relationship between eugenics and the BMI should be enough to convince any medical practitioner of the test's unsuitability, and yet it continues to be the standard around the world.

Davis' (2006) work provides a clear link between eugenics, statistics, and fatphobia. To connect these ideas to design and medical equipment requires that we consult the work of Cogdell (2003; 2010), Perez (2019), Braun (2012), and others. Work by these scholars reveals how ableism, sexism, and racism are embedded not only in our everyday materials, but especially in the medical equipment and procedures in health care practice. Cogdell (2010) argues that support for eugenics in the 1930s was at such a high that it influenced industrial designers and creators in every field:

> ...[E]volutionary and eugenic thought infiltrated American culture during this period—in the academic dream of the natural and social sciences, in theories of modern architecture, in popular culture and advertisements, in political legislation and social politics, in concerns about personal health, and in the rhetoric of speeches by industrial designers. (p. 4)

Cogdell (2003) found a "broad cultural pattern" across industries based on eugenic ideals. In researching these links, she came across a *Vogue* issue about futurism that, in part, focused on women's bodies and clothing. One designer is quoted as saying,

> Medical Science will have made her body Perfect. She'll never know "obesity," emaciation, colds in the head, superfluous hair, or a bad complexion-thanks to a controlled diet, controlled basal metabolism. Her height will be increased, her eyelashes lengthened-with some X-hormone. (Cogdell, 2003, p. 37)

In addition to influencing the conception of the acceptable human form, Cogdell (2003) found that eugenic ideology affected clothing, the telephone, lavatory equipment, train manufacturing, and even animal and livestock breeding. Material things began taking on the analogous qualities of eugenics—streamlined, progressive, unadorned, and hyper-masculine or feminine. If not always expressing a eugenic-future, designers would put materials in contrast with representations of the past—of a non-eugenic future. Materials might come off as passive, unproductive, deficient, different, and even hefty. Cogdell (2003; 2010) describes a worldview where both "man and machine" moved forward into the future, improved together by the "science" of eugenics.

Perez (2019) never fully connects her findings to eugenics, preferring instead to present readers with a mountain of historical and contemporary evidence that demonstrates a significant gender-based gap in data, in almost every field and industry. Her argument, in summary, is that the data we use to make decisions around construction, medical treatments, and even how seatbelts operate is based solely on data about men. In her discussion of medicine, Perez (2019) introduces the reader to this average man. She tells us that he is exactly 70 kg. This figure is the stand-in for all things medical—drug-testing, research examples, and practice guidelines. Men and women outside this standard have no representation and ultimately may be harmed by the significant lack of data about how their bodies work.

What Perez's gendered analysis reveals is that women have been absented as users of medical equipment. The impacts are machines, procedures, and a whole range of practices that ignore the specificity of women's bodies—including fat women. The same is true for racialized bodies. Wailoo (1997) describes the relationship between technology, disease and race as instrumental in the construction of sickle cell as an African disease. Braun (2014) focuses his analysis on spirometers—the machines created to measure lung capacities of Black slaves. He argues that the belief that race determines lung capacity is a "racial project" that arose during a time when "... instruments, measurement, and statistical analysis—increasingly reductive frameworks for understanding respiratory physiology—and problematic notions of race (p. xv)" entangled to create procedures that ultimately reduced racial difference to biology and that subsequently impacted the health outcomes of Black people throughout time. Today, spirometers are still used to measure lung capacity, but they are now race-corrected (Shaban, 2014)—an inherently flawed process of making adjustments that takes into consideration race/ethnicity (Braun et al., 2012). This history is not surprising given medicine's part in justifying the racial inferiority of Black people through scientific racism. The legacy of pseudo-science to create/explain racial difference continues still in medicine and as Vyas et al. (2020) argue, has infected the algorithms many doctors use to make critical decisions about patient treatment, including referral of specialists, use of certain drugs, and access to transplants. These include kidney function and osteoporosis risk calculators that adjust for Black versus White patients—often leading Black patients to receive better outcomes, denying them access to necessary interventions (Kolata, 2020). By examining the history of statistics, gender, and race we are witness to an exclusionary narrative that is embedded into the very architecture of medical equipment.

To put Perez (2019), Cogdell (2003; 2010), and others into conversation with one another, draws a link between statistics (or lack thereof), eugenics, and scientific racism. How we get to a place where MRI machines do not fit fat bodies becomes a little less difficult to comprehend now that we understand that for over 100 years or more, we have been designing a world away from difference and divergence. When we focus squarely on eugenics, it becomes even less difficult to see why anti-fat bias manifests in medical equipment. After all, why build equipment to accommodate a group whom we imagine always to be disappearing? The fat body is never *being* or *belonging*, but rather is always moving toward becoming less, becoming thin. Following this eugenic logic, building with inclusion in mind would ultimately be characterized as wasteful and unnecessary.

"That's a great question."

In the introduction, I describe a long list of medical equipment and devices. I could deconstruct the history and design evolution of each one of these items to determine how they impact fat patients' experiences in the health care system. However, this would take far too long and would ultimately be repetitive, given the history I outlined in the previous section. Instead, I want to focus on just one piece of equipment—MRI machines. After all, it was my doctor's comments about MRI machines and the subsequent research into MRIs that led me to write on this topic and become an accidental expert in everything MRI. As such, I think it appropriate to focus on this life-saving machine as my point of inquiry.

Although far from perfect, I must credit my family doctor for highlighting this issue. Without her remarks, flippant as they might be, I would not know that being fat meant I may never get an MRI scan. I also have to credit her for not reducing the cause of all my ailments to "obesity." This is far too common within the health care system. Many studies point to how anti-fat bias among general practitioners and within the medical field, in general, has led to subpar access to health care for fat patients (Balkhi et al., 2013; Chrisler & Barney, 2017; Lee, 2020; Persky & Eccleston, 2011; Phelan et al., 2014). Take, for example, one study where fat and non-fat patients presented with the same symptoms. The former group was advised to change parts of their lifestyle (i.e., lose weight, eat healthier, etc.), while the latter was prescribed medication (Persky & Eccleston, 2011). Chrisler and Barney (2017) make the argument that discrepancies in treatments based solely on body weight and size are a form of malpractice. Such discrepancy based solely on weight can be incredibly harmful—even deadly. As such, access to diagnostic imaging starts, not with the machine itself, but with the willingness of general practitioners to refer fat patients. It boils down to practitioners believing what we are saying.

Returning to the machine, I want to describe it in more detail to demonstrate that while its mechanics inform its shape and structure—these are not set in stone. There have been attempts to change its shape; however, even those seem to provide fat patients with more inferior options. First, a few definitions: MRI uses strong magnetic fields and radio waves to produce detailed images of the inside of the body. Nowogrodzki (2018) provides a more fulsome explanation,

> The heart of the MRI is […] a tube-like superconducting magnet, which generates a static electromagnetic field that realigns a small fraction of the hydrogen protons inside water molecules. Once those protons are lined up, coils in the scanner emit a short burst of radio-frequency waves that cause the protons' magnetic fields to wobble. When the radio burst ends, the protons release energy, sending out a faint echo of the radio waves that is detected by receiver coils and gives a picture of the anatomy …. (p. 25)

Practitioners use MRI scans to examine various parts of the body, including the brain and spinal cord, bones and joints, heart and blood vessels, breasts, and internal organs (Nowogrodzki, 2018). Understanding the mechanics of MRI machines is essential because they come in different sizes, which affects the quality of the images they produce.

The three most common types of MRI machines are closed, wide, and open bore. Closed bore machines are entirely closed and have a bore diameter between 50 and 60 cm (20–24 inches). Wide bore machines are very similar, except the bore diameter is approximately 70 cm (27.5 inches). Open bore machines are the most comfortable, having open sides and are designed with claustrophobic and fat patients in mind (Daley, n.d.). However, these machines provide lower quality images because of the position of the magnets. Closed and wide bore machines provide similar quality images, using imaging strengths between 0.5 and 3T (Tesla). Researchers in France and the United States are now conducting experimental testing with imaging strengths reaching 11.7T (Nowogrodzki, 2018). Unfortunately, the bore width for many of these new machines continues to benefit non-fat or normative bodies.

An understanding of the specifications is vital for health care practitioners because their patients may ultimately rely on them to describe the process and risks associated with using an MRI on a fat person. Practitioners should, therefore, be aware that smaller bore diameters have contributed to fat patients acquiring burns from MRI scans. These burns are a result of conduction generated through skin-to-skin contact and not from contact with the machine, although that can also be dangerous as MRI machines after long use can generate considerable heat (Gach et al., 2019). One patient acquired a thermal injury because their inner thighs were pressed against one another, thus creating "a closed loop conduction circuit" (Mandel et al., 2017, p. 349). The bore diameter, therefore, is a significant metric to keep in mind not just in determining whether the patient can fit into the machine, but also if they will be safe. Although general practitioners are not in the room when patients are scanned, they can warn their fat patients of the harm these machines pose to fat people.

Some will point to the open MRI machines as a solution to fat patients accessing imaging. However, as I argued, these provide lower quality images, and with imaging strength nearing 11.7T, no one can argue that higher-quality images are increasingly more crucial for accurate information. Still, for scans other than the brain and spine, lower-quality images produced by open bore machines would suffice. Unfortunately, these are the machines we have the fewest of in Canada. According to a 2017 report published by the Canadian Agency for Drugs and Technologies in Health, there are 366 MRI machines in 261 sites across Canada. Of the available data on 170 units, 55.3% were closed bore, 38.2% were wide bore, and only 6.5% were open bore (Sinclair et al., 2017). Data on the remaining 196 units were not available.

Additionally, there are no MRI machines in Nunavut and the Northwest Territories, and only one machine in Prince Edward Island and the Yukon (Sinclair et al., 2017). Therefore, large numbers of non-fat patients are under-served across the country, in addition to the fat patients in those provinces and territories where many Indigenous people of Canada live and already experience increased rates of prejudice and discrimination in the health care system. The solution is not more of one particular semi-capable machine. Instead, it is a reimagining of who will use these machines. More open-bore machines do not solve the issue for fat stroke or brain tumor patients who need high-quality images to ensure appropriate treatment. Fat heart-disease or lung cancer patients would also not benefit. Patients who use mobility devices, require supports to sit up, require ventilation, patients with large breasts, patients with severe claustrophobia all need a different machine, one that accommodates different sizes and different needs of various bodies. More open-bore machines would be a piecemeal solution for a problem that is system-wide, and that has a long history.

I learned a lot of the details concerning MRI machines while trying to find one that would accommodate me in my hometown of Toronto, Canada. Toronto is the largest city in Canada and is home to some of the most prominent research hospitals in the world. It was therefore utterly disappointing to learn just how inaccessible medical imaging is for fat patients. I started my search for an accessible MRI machine by doing what many people would do. I spoke with my doctor and the staff at her office. No one knew where I could get a scan. They suggested I start by calling major trauma centers as they are often the best equipped. I called the only two Level 1 centers in the Greater Toronto Area—St. Michael's Hospital and Sunnybrook Hospital. Their machines have a maximum weight of 550 pounds and a bore width of 72 centimeters.

I then did what everyone does; I Googled. My search for a list of the available MRI machines in Ontario produced no results. I decided to call the union of radiologists, hoping they would have data on the machines their members work with. Again, nothing. I decided to call Telehealth Ontario, a free, 24-hour confidential telephone service, where one can speak to and get health advice from a registered nurse. I asked the nurse on the phone about accessible MRI machines for fat patients. We discussed my case and my search for a list of the MRI machines in Ontario hospitals/medical centers. She put me on hold. Ten minutes later, she came back with nothing. She advised me to start calling hospitals directly. I called 15 hospitals and asked each about their machines.

Predictably, the capacities ranged from 400–550 pounds, with a bore width of 60, 70, and 72 cm.

Clearly, my inventory of MRI machines in Ontario is not expansive. There are over 100 hospitals in the province, and larger, more accessible machines might exist somewhere (although I would expect to find them in some of the largest hospitals in the country). In addition to bore diameter, however, my calls had uncovered another barrier—weight limitations. Hearing from technicians that many of the machines' weight limits were either below or near my weight was disconcerting. Even those with weight limitations greater than my own seemed far too close for comfort and sent a rather cold chill down my spine. Weight limits always seem to suggest an impossible figure. Picture, for example, the weight limits displayed on elevators that not only give the maximum weight (often in kilograms) but also the maximum number of occupants. This number is always ridiculously high, fanciful, and impossible (given the small spaces of most elevators). The elevator maximums, like MRI and other medical equipment (such as the CT scanners), reinforce what bodies are imagined using the equipment. For elevator manufactures, the realities of gravity, building construction, cost, etc., all limit the size and carrying capacity of their units—but I rarely come across an elevator I cannot ride. The same does not apply to MRI machines. Will not all of us need access to an MRI machine at some point in our lives? In the end, I am still unsure of what I will do when I require an MRI scan. This lack of knowledge scares me (and others; see Writer, 2020).

Before moving on to describing what I think practitioners can do to improve access to health care equipment for fat patients, I want to describe several noteworthy interactions from my calls with MRI technicians. After asking about the weight limit and bore diameter, I heard each technician say something to the effect of "That's a great question" and "Can you hold while I check?" These responses were somehow simultaneously validating and worrying. The first response is validating because it suggests that such information should be made available and is important for a small but equally significant group in society. It is "a great question" because the machine may be too small for some individuals. However, taking the responses together, I worry that technicians have to check. This suggests technicians rarely get asked about the specifications of their machines, which sadly confirms the research that fat patients may be receiving other diagnostic/treatment plans that purposefully avoid MRI scans.

I want to discuss one final noteworthy interaction. After confirming my weight and height, one technician proceeded to make assumptions about where I "hold my weight" and how my height inferred an equal weight distribution and, therefore, a better chance of fitting into the machine. Their logic is not sound. Height does not guarantee equal proportionality in size or weight distribution. Their comments draw me back to Galton's preference for tallness and how my imagined tall, fat body, for this technician was more proportional than a short, fat body. What this interaction underscores is who we imagine will use this equipment. It is certainly not anyone close to the weight limit or whose girth matches the bore diameter, and it is certainly not anyone who is disproportionate, disabled, disfigured, has a large chest, and/or a large rear. The normative imagined figure whom we build these machines for is reflective of the logic created by eugenics—the norm, the average man, the non-disabled. We unconsciously hold this figure up, even though they do not exist, and never existed. We base so much of our material things on this composite that we end up creating products that exclude large numbers of the population.

The zoo or a new industry

It seems, for now, that the solution to this problem continues to be the open-bore MRI machines. Other solutions include a somewhat controversial use of non-human MRI machines for fat patients. In both Australia and the United Kingdom, doctors have sent their fat patients to local animal hospitals or zoos for scans (Adams, 2012; Meikle, 2013). Reports on this phenomenon simultaneously fat-shame patients and evoke sympathy from readers. However, they also, unexpectedly, expose the eugenic logics that underscore manufacturing of "for human" medical equipment that enforces an average or normative size of human. There are other arguments to be made about an anthropocentric worldview that divides humans and animals. The harm that comes with having fat people use the same machines as animals stems less from whom we are sharing them with, and more so from the knowledge that animals (and thus fat bodies) are disposable in our society. Russell and Semenko (2016) describe this as "fatness as animalized" and suggest that the result is the abjection of both fat and animal bodies.

The zoo might be one solution, especially if the imaging strength is strong. Another solution stems from the manufactories of medical equipment. Although there are no reports for a fat-specific closed/wide MRI machine, "bariatric" products are a growing industry that make up nearly 10% of some company's sales (Morgans, 2014). While it is significant that manufacturers are finally committing resources to develop these products, they are only responding to demands by medical staff and the willingness of governments and hospitals to purchase fat-specific equipment. Allocating more resources to making medical spaces—all of them, and not merely "bariatric-specific" units—accessible is excellent news to many of us.

I do worry, however, about the fatting of medical equipment as an ultimately capitalist endeavor that fails to address the underlying eugenic logic that led us to construct a world for figures that do not exist. We might be making bigger beds for fat patients, but I also wonder about who else benefits from a larger bed, a wider chair, grab bars in the bathroom, and lifts in hospital rooms and surgery theatres. Can we imagine "bariatric-sized" furniture being utilized by non-fat people—a parent desperate to sit close to their adult child, siblings sitting side-by-side, an older patient independently showering, and a physically disabled person having more access to medical spaces? We may be building for fat people, but I do not think fat people should be the only users of this equipment. Maybe building a larger, more durable, wider MRI machine might benefit all of us and not just fat folks. However, if it did only benefits fat folks, its constructions should still be worthwhile.

At the beginning of this piece, I stated that in the course of trying to find an MRI machine that would fit me, I became an accidental expert. Becoming an expert takes a lot of time. Taking that time—calling, researching, and writing this piece—is something that I should not have to do to get an MRI scan. I have put far too much labor in trying to produce access for myself. I want to make this labor the responsibility of medical practitioners.

To make your practice more accessible for fat bodies, I would encourage you to review the list of medical equipment and devices in the first paragraph of this piece. Then, audit your office and consider if a fat person can fit and would be comfortable in the space. For devices and equipment outside a general practitioner's office, such as an MRI machine or CT scanner, consider finding out which devices in your area would accommodate fat patients. Consult with other doctors and staff. Ask local representatives. Ask fat patients about their experiences and see what knowledge they have amassed. Keep this information handy. Share it with others and update it as new information becomes available. Do not stop with just equipment, however, but consider new procedures with those devices. Draw blood from a patient's hand, instead of their elbows (especially if you cannot find a vein in the elbow crease). Instruct patients to take care when using MRI machines, and about the dangers of skin-to skin-contact. Use wrist blood pressure cuffs instead of the traditional arm cuffs. And most importantly, believe your fat patients and be open to new ways of producing care.

Finally, consider consulting with other professionals—dentists, occupational therapists, physical therapists—about techniques they use to accommodate fat patients. Do research. Keep up to date on medical advancements, but also consult other sources, such as the following journals: *Fat Studies, Body & Society,* and *Body Image: An International Journal of Research* and blogs, Dances with Fat and The Body is Not an Apology. You might also consider following fat people on social media (scholars, artists, activists, musicians, actors, etc.) and seeing them live their lives fully. If nothing else, try to dislodge the image of the average person from your mind and work actively to embrace the multiplicity of who is out there and should be included.

References

Adams, S. (2012, November 1). *Obesity crisis "will force hospitals to use super-size MRI scanners at zoos."* https://www.telegraph.co.uk/news/health/news/9649738/Obesity-crisis-will-force-hospitals-to-use-super-size-MRI-scanners-at-zoos.html

Amy, N. K., Aalborg, A., Lyons, P., & Keranen, L. (2006). Barriers to routine gynecological cancer screening for White and African-American obese women. *International Journal of Obesity, 30*(1), 147. https://doi.org/10.1038/sj.ijo.0803105

Balkhi, A. M., Parent, M. C., & Mayor, M. (2013). Impact of perceived weight discrimination on patient satisfaction and physician trust. *Fat Studies, 2*(1), 45–55. https://doi.org/10.1080/21604851.2013.731955

Braun, L. (2014). *Breathing race into the machine: The surprising career of the spirometer from plantation to genetics.* University of Minnesota Press.

Braun, L., Wolfgang, M., & Dickersin, K. (2012). Defining race/ethnicity and explaining difference in research studies on lung function. *European Respiratory Journal, 41*, 1362–1370. https://doi.org/10.1183/09031936.00091612

Chrisler, J. C., & Barney, A. (2017). Sizeism is a health hazard. *Fat Studies, 6*(1), 38–53. https://doi.org/10.1080/21604851.2016.1213066

Cogdell, C. (2003). Products or bodies? Streamline design and eugenics as applied biology. *Design Issues, 19*(1), 36–53.

Cogdell, C. (2010). *Eugenic design: Streamlining America in the 1930s.* University of Pennsylvania Press.

Daley, B. (n.d.). *3 types of MRI machines and the difference between an open MRI vs. a closed MRI.* https://4rai.com/blog/3-types-of-mri-machines

Davis, L. J. (2006). Constructing normalcy: The bell curve, the novel, and the invention of the disabled body in the nineteenth century. In L. J. Davis (Ed.), *The disability studies reader* (2nd ed., pp. 3–16). Routledge.

Diconsiglio, J. (2006). Hospitals equip to meet the bariatric challenge. Rising number of obese patients necessitates specific supplies. *Materials Management in Health Care, 15*(4), 36–39.

Eknoyan, G. (2007). Adolphe Quetelet (1796–1874) the average man and indices of obesity. *Nephrology Dialysis Transplantation, 23*(1), 47–51. https://doi.org/10.1093/ndt/gfm517

Gach, H. M., Mackey, S. L., Hausman, S. E., Jackson, D. R., Benzinger, T. L., Henke, L., Murphy, L. A., Fluchel, J. L., Cai, B., Zoberi, J. E., Garcia-Ramirez, J., Mutic, S., & Schwarz, J. K. (2019). MRI safety risks in the obese: The case of the disposable lighter stored in the pannus. *Radiology Case Reports, 14*(5), 634–638. https://doi.org/10.1016/j.radcr.2019.02.023

Garland-Thomson, R. (1997). *Extraordinary bodies: Figuring physical disability in American culture and literature.* Columbia University Press.

Kaminsky, J., & Gadaleta, D. (2002). A study of discrimination within the medical community as viewed by obese patients. *Obesity Surgery, 12*(1), 14–18. https://doi.org/10.1381/096089202321144513

Kolata, G. (2020, July 21). Many medical decision tools disadvantage Black patients. *The New York Times.* https://www.nytimes.com/2020/06/17/health/many-medical-decision-tools-disadvantage-black-patients.html

Lee, J. (2020). "You will face discrimination": Fatness, motherhood, and the medical profession. *Fat Studies, 9*(1), 1–16. https://doi.org/10.1080/21604851.2019.1595289

Mandel, N. S., Ramdial, J. L., & Marcus, E. N. (2017). A second-degree burn after MRI. *Cleveland Clinic Journal of Medicine, 84*(5), 348–349. https://doi.org/10.3949/ccjm.84a.15164

Meikle, J. (2013, May 17). Scanner scandal: Are zoos using animal equipment on obese humans? *The Guardian.* https://www.theguardian.com/society/blog/2013/may/17/scanner-zoos-equipment-animals-obese

Merrill, E., & Grassley, J. (2008). Women's stories of their experiences as overweight patients. *Journal of Advanced Nursing, 64*(2), 139–146. https://doi.org/10.1111/j.1365-2648.2008.04794.x

Mitchell, D., & Snyder, S. (2003). The eugenic Atlantic: Race, disability, and the making of an international eugenic science, 1800–1945. *Disability & Society, 18*(7), 843–864.

Morgans, J. (2014, June 19). Fat-people medical equipment is on the cusp of a boom. *Vice.* https://www.vice.com/en_au/article/vdpzkb/fat-people-medical-equipment-is-on-the-cusp-of-a-boom

Nowogrodzki, A. (2018). The world's strongest MRI machines are pushing human imaging to new limits. *Nature, 563*(7729), 24–26. https://doi.org/10.1038/d41586-018-07182-7

Perez, C. C. (2019). *Invisible women: Exposing data bias in a world designed for men.* Random House.

Persky, S., & Eccleston, C. P. (2011). Medical student bias and care recommendations for an obese versus non-obese virtual patient. *International Journal of Obesity, 35*(5), 728–735. https://doi.org/10.1038/ijo.2010.173

Phelan, S. M., Dovidio, J. F., Puhl, R. M., Burgess, D. J., Nelson, D. B., Yeazel, M. W., Hardeman, R., Perry, S., & van Ryn, M. (2014). Implicit and explicit weight bias in a national sample of 4,732 medical students: The medical student CHANGES study. *Obesity, 22*(4), 1201–1208. https://doi.org/10.1002/oby.20687

Phelan, S. M., Burgess, D. J., Yeazel, M. W., Hellerstedt, W. L., Griffin, J. M., & van Ryn, M. (2015). Impact of weight bias and stigma on quality of care and outcomes for patients with obesity: Obesity stigma and patient care. *Obesity Reviews, 16*(4), 319–326. https://doi.org/10.1111/obr.12266

Pryor, W. (2002). The health care disadvantages of being obese. *New South Wales Public Health Bulletin, 13*(7), 163–165. https://doi.org/10.1071/NB02066

Russell, C. L., & Semenko, K. (2016). We take "cow" as a compliment: Fattening humane, environmental, and social justice education. In E. Cameron & C. Russell (Eds.), *The fat pedagogy reader: Challenging weight-based oppression through critical pedagogy* (pp. 211–220). Peter Lang.

Shaban, H. (2014, August 29). How racism creeps into medicine. *The Atlantic.* https://www.theatlantic.com/health/archive/2014/08/how-racism-creeps-into-medicine/378618/

Sinclair, A., Morrison, A., Young, C., & Pyke, L. (2017). *Canadian Medical Imaging Inventory, 2017.* Canadian Agency for Drugs and Technologies in Health.

Vyas, D. A., Eisenstein, L. G., & Jones, D. S. (2020). Hidden in plain sight—Reconsidering the use of race correction in clinical algorithms. *New England Journal of Medicine, 383*(9), 874–882. https://doi.org/10.1056/NEJMms2004740

Wann, M. (2009). Foreword: Fat studies: An invitation to revolution. In E. Rothblum & S. Solovay (Eds.), *The fat studies reader* (pp. ix–xxv). New York University Press.

Wailoo, K. (1997). *Drawing blood: Technology and disease identity in twentieth-century America.* Jhu Press.

Writer, J. J. (2020, February 20). This is what life is really like when you weigh over 400 pounds. *HuffPost.* https://www.huffpost.com/entry/infinifat-fat-life-over-400-pounds-fatphobia_n_5e4ad05bc5b64ba297534c7c

4 "Limited by body habitus"

Fat and stigmatizing rhetoric in medical records

Jennifer Renee Blevins

The first time I saw the phrase "limited by body habitus" in my father's medical records, I probably cocked my head and furrowed my brow, but didn't think too much of it. After the third or fourth instance, I Googled the term "body habitus" and discovered that it meant exactly what I thought it meant: "the physique or body build" of a patient (Shiel, n.d.). Therefore, "limited by body habitus" means that a patient's body limits an exam or procedure, thereby shifting the blame for incomplete or inadequate medical treatment from the doctor to the patient. In other words, every time the medical professionals who recorded my father's ordeal believed that his fat body prevented them from treating his fat body, they wrote, "limited by body habitus." They wrote it over two dozen times.

On March 24, 2010, my father had a routine gastric bypass procedure in Durham, North Carolina, that went catastrophically wrong. He spent over a year in ICUs, hospitals, and rehab facilities and had more than 20 surgeries to contend with the consequences of that initial surgery. I moved from New York City to North Carolina to take care of him during this period, and in the years that followed I wrote a book about the experience. Part memoir, part cultural analysis, *Limited by Body Habitus: An American Fat Story* (Blevins, 2019) details the experience of serving as my father's advocate and caretaker and investigates the history of fat stigma in the United States. Bringing together experiences of personal and national trauma, I weave the tale of my father's botched gastric bypass surgery and subsequent prolonged health crisis with the environmental catastrophe of the Deepwater Horizon oil spill. These intertwined narratives, both disasters that could have been avoided, reveal points of failure in our systems of health care and environmental conservation. Incorporating excerpts from medical records, journal entries, news stories, government documents, and other sources, I complicate the dominant discourse surrounding the "obesity epidemic" as I tell the story of my family, our bodies, and our very American history with fat.

In what follows, I will draw from my book and my work as a literature and Fat Studies scholar to address fat bias in the medical industry and provide a critical perspective for pedagogy and practice. I aim to problematize the dominant rhetoric surrounding fat patients and offer alternative methods for chronicling

DOI: 10.4324/9781003057000-5

the experiences of diverse bodies in health care settings. I will discuss how I utilize Mikhail Bakhtin's (1981) concept of heteroglossia in my book to both convey the fragmentary, un-representable nature of trauma and to problematize and decentralize the "unitary language" employed by the medical practitioners who chronicled my father's lengthy hospitalization. Moreover, I will consider the ways in which the language of the medical records inflicts additional trauma by rendering my fat father "hyper(in)visible" (Gailey, 2014). This chapter will argue that future and current health care providers must consider their patients not only physiologically but *rhetorically* as well. In other words, medical practitioners should be educated regarding how language constructs a subject, and how phrases like "limited by body habitus" frame fat patients as obstacles and negatively influence the way that health care providers approach those patients.

Confronting my own stigma

As I discuss in my book, when my father had his gastric bypass surgery in 2010, I was a staunch believer in the inherent dangers of fat, and it was not until I commenced my research for the project that would become *Limited by Body Habitus* that I began to question my beliefs. I made troubling discoveries, like the fact that the National Institutes of Health's decision to lower body mass index (BMI) levels in 1998—a change that made millions of Americans "overweight" or "obese" literally overnight—was significantly influenced by the work of the International Obesity Task Force, whose members had direct financial ties to pharmaceutical companies that manufactured diet pills for profit (Moynihan, 2006; Squires, 1998). From J. Eric Oliver's (2006) *Fat Politics: The Real Story Behind America's Obesity Epidemic*, I learned that the BMI chart—the American Medical Association's primary tool for diagnosing "obesity"—was created by a Belgian astronomer in the 1830s, not a doctor practicing modern-day medicine, and that the two studies published in the *Journal of the American Medical Association* in the 1990s that effectively kicked off the "war on obesity" utilized questionable methodology, such as attributing the deaths of all "obese" people to their fat, even if they had died from a snakebite or a car crash.[1] In my research, I also discovered that some physicians, such as Katherine M. Flegal (Flegal et al., 2013), Sandra Aamodt (2016), and Carl Lavie (2014), have challenged widely accepted beliefs in the medical industry regarding the correlation between "obesity" and mortality rates, while scholars like Amy Erdmann Farrell (2011) and Sabrina Strings (2019) have examined the fraught relationships between fatness, race, and citizenship. Similar to Oliver and Farrell, who both admit in the prefaces of their books that the discoveries they made when researching their topic changed their view of fat and thus altered the focus of their projects, the research for *Limited by Body Habitus* radically transformed my writing process, because it opened my eyes to the fact that the "truth" about fat was much more complicated than the discourse surrounding the "obesity epidemic" claims.

In retrospect, it shouldn't have taken years of research for me to question my beliefs about fat, since I witnessed so many examples of the medical industry's bias toward fat patients firsthand during the year that I cared for my father after his botched gastric bypass. Before doctors realized that my father had developed a leak between his new stomach pouch and esophagus, one of the bariatric surgeons admonished him for not getting out of his hospital bed to walk, even though he told them that walking caused him great pain. After my father became septic with multiple organ failure and was hooked up to a ventilator in the ICU, I heard through a hospital social worker that there were rumors that he had caused his own leak by engaging in "noncompliant" behavior. When I began the research for my book, I found studies that prove the ways in which many medical practitioners are biased against fat patients, thus confirming my father's experience (see Foster et al., 2003; Phelan et al., 2014; Phelan et al., 2015; Schwartz et al., 2003). More than half of the 620 primary-care doctors in one of the studies "viewed 'obese' patients as awkward, unattractive, ugly, and noncompliant" (Foster et al., 2003, p. 1168). Disturbingly (but perhaps not surprisingly), even medical professionals who specialize in treating "obesity" exhibit implicit and explicit bias toward fat patients. Schwartz et al. (2003) determined that the "obesity specialists" in their research sample "associated the stereotypes lazy, stupid, and worthless with 'obese' people," even though the group was comprised of practitioners who understood that "obesity is caused by genetic and environmental factors and is not simply a function of individual behavior" (p. 1037). These findings and my initial failure to recognize my own confirmation bias illustrate the extent to which we internalize fat hatred so deeply that it can be hard to acknowledge, even when confronted with evidence that directly contradicts our beliefs.

One of the primary ways that the medical industry perpetuates this fat stigma is through the language that clinicians use to describe fat patients. According to Goddu et al. (2018), exposure to stigmatizing language in medical records is associated with more negative attitudes toward patients and less aggressive management of a patient's pain. In fact, the study found that physicians-in-training can internalize the implicit bias in medical notes that have been written by their seniors and peers, a phenomenon which the authors of the study refer to as "part of the 'hidden curriculum' of medical training" (Goddu et al., 2018, p. 685). Since other medical professionals, such as social workers, nurses, physical therapists, and dieticians, are expected to follow the lead of the physician, the effects of this "hidden curriculum" can trickle down and influence every stratum of the health care field. The fact that some of this stigmatizing language (like "limited by body habitus") is common parlance in the medical industry suggests that the root of the bias is not only personal but institutional. In other words, regardless of their personal implicit or explicit bias, medical students are taught to rhetorically construct fat patients in stigmatizing ways. Historically speaking, the medical gaze has not been kind to fat people.

Early in my writing process, I asked my father to request copies of his medical records. I had intended to use the records to simply help me recreate the events of that year with greater accuracy, but once I started reading them I was struck by some of the language used to describe my father. I write about this experience in a chapter titled "I See Fat People":

> When I read through the language used in my father's medical records, I can tell that the authors see his body, but they also don't see it. His fat body is often depicted as a barrier or obstacle to overcome. Many of the health professionals who chronicled my father's story seem oblivious to the power of language, to the detrimental effect that word choice can have on real lives. Even when they appear to compliment him they do him a disservice; the repeated insistence on how 'pleasant' the 'obese white male' in the bed is paints my father as a sort of Santa Claus—jolly and likable, in spite of his fat. Also, the emphasis on his 'whiteness' in the medical records makes me wonder how differently he might have been perceived (and treated) if he had been a person of color, instead of a 'pleasant' old white man. (Blevins, 2019, pp. 136–137)

When I write that the practitioners who authored my father's medical records "see his body, but they also don't see it," I am identifying a phenomenon referred to as "hyper(in)visibility" (Gailey, 2014). Gailey argues that fat presents a paradox, because fat people are both "hypervisible" and "hyperinvisible": "To be hyper(in) visible means that a person is sometimes paid exceptional attention and is sometimes exceptionally overlooked, and it can happen simultaneously" (p. 7). The repeated mentions of my father's "morbid obesity" and the "limits" of his body in the medical records demonstrate the paradox of hyper(in)visibility by illustrating how the clinicians perceived his body size and its "limitations" as central to both his identity and his maladies, yet seemed blind to the ways that their bias had circumscribed his identity while completely omitting the fact that their failures had limited (and almost killed) his body. Therefore, creatively integrating the medical records into my book became a recuperative and subversive act, because doing so helped me combat this hyper(in)visibility by presenting two different versions of my father's story—the visceral, lived experience of the tragedy, versus the official, "objective" account, in which phrases like "limited by body habitus" portray my father's fat body as inconvenient and noncompliant.

Some clinicians may not understand why "limited by body habitus" is so stigmatizing, especially when applied to a fat patient. Since, as Goddu et al. (2018) establish in their study, physicians absorb the bias of their mentors and peers, they may never stop to question the appropriateness of stigmatizing terms such as "overweight," for example (which is problematic because it implies that there is a "normal" weight that everyone must strive to achieve, regardless of the realities of bodily diversity). I imagine that most clinicians read medical records solely as a description of a patient's medical history, since their job is treating the patient's illness. As a literature scholar and creative writer, however, I studied my father's medical records as a text to interpret and evaluate, focusing on literary elements like tone, word choice, and figurative language, and considered the ways in which my father's body is a socially constructed projection, not merely the raw material for medical procedures. For instance, the repetition of the phrase "limited by body habitus" brought to mind French sociologist Pierre Bourdieu's (1984) concept of "habitus," which is a term for our social environment and the commodities we surround ourselves with to project a certain class identity, as well as the way that culture and personal experiences shape the body and mind. Habitus structures and organizes our perception of the social world, because it determines the way that we internalize class divisions. Since, as Bourdieu states, "social identity is defined and asserted through difference," habitus constitutes the identity of the individuals we encounter, for we make value judgments based on their different mannerisms, tastes, attitudes, and appearance (p. 172). These judgments affect lives, because, as Bourdieu explains, habitus is "the basis of an alchemy which transforms the distribution of capital, the balance-sheet of a power relation, into a system of perceived differences, distinctive properties, that is, a distribution of symbolic capital, legitimate capital, whose objective truth is misrecognized" (p. 172). That is, habitus influences power relations between individuals, because the differences that we perceive in others determine social positions. Therefore, reading my father's medical records through the lens of Bourdieu's concept of "habitus" offers one way of illustrating the stigmatizing nature of the phrase "limited by body habitus": proclaiming that habitus "limits" my father effectively relegates him to the lower rungs of a social hierarchy, rendering him a liability on the "balance-sheet of a power relation." This power dynamic reflects the general consensus of our fat hating society, in which "fat people are often treated as *not quite human*, entities to whom the normal standards of polite and respectful behavior do not seem to apply" (Farrell, 2011, p. 6). Thus, while clinicians view terminology like "limited by body habitus" as benign descriptors, a critical close reading can reveal the stigma inherent in their rhetoric.

Challenging medically-biased language

Part of my project in *Limited by Body Habitus: An American Fat Story* was to find a way to help the reader (and, hopefully, future health care workers) to really *see* a fat patient—to humanize and give voice to a patient who might otherwise be dismissed and marginalized based on their body size. Additionally, I wanted to recreate the events of that year in such a way that conveyed the fragmentary, unrepresentable nature of trauma. To accomplish these goals, I utilized a non-linear, experimental form, emphasizing heteroglossia.

Russian philosopher Mikhail Bakhtin's concept of heteroglossia translates from the Greek to "different tongues," or "different languages." In his original 1934 paper "Discourse in the Novel," Bakhtin draws a distinction between unitary language and heteroglossia. He explains that unitary language is "a system of linguistic norms" that attempts to unify and centralize ideology and language (1934/1981, p. 270). For instance, medical records may be viewed as an example of unitary language. Heteroglossia, on the other hand, he defines as, "*another's speech in another's language,* serving to express authorial intentions but in a refracted way" (Bakhtin, 1934/1981, p. 270). In other words, heteroglossia involves the use of multiple voices in a text to convey the author's ideas. (One famous literary example of this technique is T.S. Eliot's poem "The Waste Land.") Unitary language seeks to suppress heteroglossia, because it threatens to rupture the façade of cohesion and centralization that unitary language strives to present.

In my book, I challenge the "unitary language" of the medical records through my use of heteroglossia. The main narrative often engages with the institutional narrative presented in my father's medical records, at times in a dialogic manner. For instance, in the chapter "Medical Records Medley," the speaker directly responds to the rhetoric in the medical records. As her frustration and anger with her father's unresolved leak grow, so do her frustration and anger with the use of stigmatizing phrases like "limited by body habitus." By the end of the chapter, the speaker attempts to reason with voice of the medical records:

EXAMINATION: 7103 – CXR PORTABLE EXAM Apr 26 2010

REASON: RESPIRATORY DISTRESS

Study is limited by body habitus. Depth of inspiration is shallow … Increasing bilateral airspace disease consistent with pneumonia or atelectasis.

You see, here's the thing: we are all limited by body habitus. The fragile, leaky, mushy, mortal body is the one limitation we all share. Those tired, labored lungs in my father's chest that are collapsing and inflamed and filling with fluid, those are your lungs, too. The act of breathing, currently compromised by those failing lungs, is necessary for your survival, too. The pierceable skin, the delicate tissue, the breakable bones, the fickle organs, the susceptible brain—all limiting, all aspects of being alive.

You say that your study of my father's body is limited by my father's body. No, my father is limited by his body, as you are by yours. Your study is limited because the medical industry has long privileged certain body types when designing tests, procedures, equipment, and education. This limitation exemplifies a history of fat discrimination that follows us even here—to a hospital that specializes in weight loss surgery for the morbidly obese. Your study is limited because the way that the medical community perceives fat bodies has been limited. My father's body is simply my father's body—finite, precarious, and loved. (Blevins, 2019, pp. 74–75)

Throughout "Medical Records Medley," the voice of the speaker challenges the authority of the medical records, thereby undermining their centrality.

My application of heteroglossia also provided the opportunity to include my father's voice. Because I kept notes and journals throughout the experience, I was able to use exact quotes from conversations that he and I had during his hospitalization. In one chapter, "Moving, Part One," the writing style suddenly shifts from prose to play dialogue, as I pull the reader into a conversation we had one night after a traumatizing experience, during a period when his mental status was severely altered. Other "voices" that I incorporate into the book include personal journal entries, news stories, government documents, derogatory online comments posted to a story about "obesity," and segments of literary works that I recited to my father while he was in the hospital. The different voices collide in the epilogue, which puts the medical records in conversation with the main narrative voice and the other voices that have appeared throughout the book. By depicting my father's medical disaster as a polyphonic mosaic, rather than as a linear narrative told by a singular voice, Limited by Body Habitus attempts to unsettle and complicate the reader's preconceived notions of both trauma and fat.

Recommendations

To stop perpetuating implicit and explicit fat bias, medical professionals must reevaluate the ways that they talk and write about fat patients. This undertaking would necessitate an examination of the bias of individual practitioners as well as the stigmatizing rhetoric that is currently commonplace in the medical industry. I propose beginning this process by developing methods by which physicians-in-training may come to know and perceive fat people as individuals with their own stories, rather than as "noncompliant" patients that they must "fix." In addition to critically reexamining the language used in medical records to describe fat patients, I recommend expanding the process of documenting interactions with patients to include Rita Charon's (2006) concept of the "Parallel Chart" (p. 149).

In Narrative Medicine: Honoring the Stories of Illness, Charon (2006) acknowledges the power of the terminology that physicians use to describe patients and cautions against inadvertently blaming patients for their health problems:

> Such descriptions as "morbidly obese" and "sexually promiscuous" transform a physical or behavioral description into not only a moral judgment of the patient but also an accusation that the patient caused whatever ails her ... [which] gives the doctor an excuse in failing to cure disease. (p. 31)

One of the founders of the field of narrative medicine, Charon (2006) proposes that medical practitioners should engage in reflective writing activities about their interactions with patients that allow them to include "the 'I' of the writing subject" (p. 149). She describes the idea of a "Parallel Chart," which is not restricted by the conventions of official medical records, as "writing done in nontechnical language that captures the personal and metaphorical dimensions of meaning, both for the sick person and those caring for the sick person" (Charon, 2006, p. 149). In other words, Charon recommends that clinicians write creatively and reflectively about their experiences with patients. Similar to my use of heteroglossia in Limited by Body Habitus, these writings would problematize the unitary language of the medical records by supplementing and possibly even engaging with them in a dialogic manner. While not part of the official medical record, this "Parallel Chart" could serve as a forum for acknowledging and working through implicit and explicit bias toward fat patients. Also, by focusing on the patient's narrative, as well as reflecting on the narrative that unfolds between caregiver and patient, clinicians may be more likely to perceive their fat patients as complex, vulnerable individuals, rather than as "noncompliant" obstacles. Particularly important for physicians-in-training, this practice of humanizing fat patients through narrative competence could be the first step toward decreasing stigmatizing rhetoric about diverse bodies in the medical industry.

Ten years ago, as I sat in an ICU and watched a machine breathe for my father, the fear I felt was matched only by my rage. Some mysterious medical mishap had abruptly transformed my intelligent, witty father into a comatose, critically ill body in a bed, and for months I watched powerlessly as various health care professionals tended to him without really seeing him. I felt compelled to tell them my father's story—to encourage them to see past their implicit weight bias by humanizing the 350-pound body that they had been charged with keeping alive. In at least one instance, I succeeded. When one of the bariatric fellows visited my father's ICU room on the last day of his rotation, he thanked me and said, "Your father's case has been a profound learning experience for me." As moved as I was by his words at the time, I now realize that my father and I should not have been the ones teaching this surgical fellow to care about fat people. Such an intervention needs to begin during the first year of medical school, where an anti-bias education should be part of the standard curriculum. Doctors must learn that words matter—that their rhetorical choices can be as crucial as their medical decisions, because stigmatizing language can have devastating consequences for their patients.

Note

1 The two studies that commenced the "war on obesity" are Allison, D. B., Fontain, K. R., Manson, J. E., Stevens, J., & VanItallie, T. (1999). Annual deaths attributable to obesity in the United States. *Journal of the American Medical Association, 282*(16), 1530–1538 and Mokdad, A. H., Marks, J. S., Stroup, D. F., & Gerberding, J. I. (2004). Actual causes of death in the United States, 2000. *Journal of the American Medical Association, 291*(10), 1238–1245. Oliver notes that "in neither of these studies did the researchers actually measure the linkage between obesity and death" (Oliver, 2006, p. 24).

References

Aamodt, S. (2016). *Why diets make us fat: The unintended consequences of our obsession with weight loss.* Scribe.

Bakhtin, M. (1981). Discourse in the novel (C. Emerson, Trans.). In C. Emerson & M. Holquist (Eds.), *The dialogic imagination: Four essays.* University of Texas Press. (Original work published 1934.)

Blevins, J. R. (2019). *Limited by body habitus: An American fat story.* Autumn House Press.

Bourdieu, P. (1984). *Distinction: A social critique of the judgement of taste* (R. Nice, Trans.). Harvard University Press.

Charon, R. (2006). *Narrative medicine: Honoring the stories of illness.* Oxford University Press.

Farrell, A. E. (2011). *Fat shame: Stigma and the fat body in American culture.* New York University Press.

Flegal, K. M., Kit, B. K., Orpana, H., & Graubard, B. I. (2013). Association of all-cause mortality with overweight and obesity using standard body mass index categories: A systematic review and meta-analysis. *Journal of the American Medical Association*, 309(1), 71–82. https://doi.org.10.1001/jama.2012.113905

Foster, G. D., Wadden, T. A., Makris, A. P., Davidson, D., Sanderson, R. S., Allison, D. B., & Kessler, A. (2003). Primary care physicians' attitudes about obesity and its treatment. *Obesity Research*, 11(10), 1168–1177. https://doi.org/10.1038/oby.2003.161

Gailey, J. A. (2014). *The hyper(in)visible fat woman: Weight and gender discourse in contemporary society*. Palgrave Macmillan.

Goddu, A. P., O'Conor, K. J., Lanzkron, S., Saheed, M. O., Saha, S., Peek, M. E., Haywood, C., Jr., & Beach, M. C. (2018). Do words matter? Stigmatizing language and the transmission of bias in the medical record. *Journal of General Internal Medicine*, 33(5), 685–691. https://doi.org/10.1007/s11606-017-4289-2

Lavie, C. J. (2014). *The obesity paradox: When thinner means sicker and heavier means healthier*. Penguin.

Moynihan, R. (2006). Obesity task force linked to WHO takes "millions" from drug firms. *British Medical Journal*, 332, 1412. https://doi.org/10.1136/bmj.332.7555.1412-a

Oliver, J. E. (2006). *Fat politics: The real story behind America's obesity epidemic*. Oxford University Press.

Phelan, S. M., Burgess, D. J., Yeazel, M. W., Hellerstedt, W. L., Griffin, J. M., & van Ryn, M. (2015). Impact of weight bias and stigma on quality of care and outcomes for patients with obesity. *Obesity Reviews*, 16(4), 319–326. https://doi.org/10.1111/obr.12266

Phelan, S. M., Dovidio, J. F., Puhl, R. M., Burgess, D. J., Nelson, D. B., Yeazel, M. W., Hardeman, R., Perry, S., & Van Ryn, M. (2014). Implicit and explicit weight bias in a national sample of 4,732 medical students: The medical student CHANGES study. *Obesity*, 22(4), 1201–1208. https://doi.org/10.1002/oby.20687

Schwartz, M. B., Chambliss, H. O. N., Brownell, K. D., Blair, S. N., & Billington, C. (2003). Weight bias among health professionals specializing in obesity. *Obesity Research*, 11(9), 1033–1039. https://doi.org/10.1038/oby.2003.142

Shiel, W. C. (n.d.). Medical definition of body habitus. *MedicineNet*. https://www.medicinenet.com/script/main/art.asp?articlekey=21671

Squires, S. (1998, June 4). Optimal weight threshold lowered. *Washington Post*. https://www.washingtonpost.com/archive/politics/1998/06/04/optimal-weight-threshold-lowered/a1226b77-2726-4e40-9161-b7643cd539f9/

Strings, S. (2019). *Fearing the Black body: The racial origins of fat phobia*. New York University Press.

5 "God forbid you bring a cupcake"

Theorizing biopedagogies as professional socialization in dietetics education

Meredith Bessey and Jennifer Brady

According to the International Confederation of Dietetic Associations (2014), dietitians are "professional[s] who appl[y] the science of food and nutrition to promote health, [and] prevent and treat disease to optimize the health of individuals, groups, communities and populations" (para. 3). When viewed through the lens of formal education and training, as well as licensure requirements, becoming a dietitian means demonstrating mastery in the knowledge and therapeutic application of food, nutrition, and health science. In Canada, securing licensure to practice dietetics requires that students complete a 4-year undergraduate degree that is accredited by Dietitians of Canada, as well as an internship of about 48 weeks, after which hopefuls write a standardized licensing exam (the Canadian Dietetic Registration Examination). Securing an internship is highly competitive with a success rate of less than half, which leaves many unable to complete their training (Siswanto et al., 2015). Ruhl and Lordly (2017) report that a culture of competition pervades dietetics education as a result of the internship application and selection process. Others have observed that dietetics education is dominated by a positivist, biomedical paradigm of food, nutrition, health, and the body (Aphramor & Gingras, 2009; Fraser & Brady, 2018; Gingras & Brady, 2010), which has been particularly evident in the profession's fat oppressive focus on the prevention, management, and treatment of "obesity."

Beyond the precepts of formal education and training, becoming a dietitian is also a matter of professional socialization (Lordly & MacLellan, 2012; MacLellan et al., 2011). Goldenberg and Iwasiw (1993) define professional socialization as

> a complex and interactive process by which the content of the professional role (skills, knowledge, behavior) is learned and the values, attitudes, and goals integral to the profession and sense of occupational identity which are characteristic of a member of that profession are internalized. (p. 4)

Yet, dietitian-scholars have noted that the process of becoming professional extends even farther than students' cognitive and affective states, to commandeer their corporeal selves. That is, becoming a dietitian is an embodied process whereby the dietitian body comes to stand as testament to their mastery of

DOI: 10.4324/9781003057000-6

professional knowledge and authority, as well as professional identity and belong-ingness (Brady, 2018; Gingras & Brady, 2010). Some have sardonically noted that being thin is a "professional credential" of good dietitians (e.g., Brady, 2018; Gingras & Brady, 2010; Rochefort et al., 2016; Schaeffer, 2014). Yet, there has been little work to date that theorizes professional socialization as an embodied process, and no work that explores professional socialization *vis a vis* fat oppres-sion and health professions education.

This chapter seeks to theorize the interface of professional socialization and biopedagogies in the context of post-secondary health professions education, spe-cifically the education and training of dietitians. Briefly, biopedagogies is a con-cept rooted in Foucauldian notions of biopower and disciplinary power. Wright and Halse (2014) describe biopedagogies as "the values and practices that are disseminated through informal education (e.g., media and Internet) as well as formal education (e.g., school) which work to instruct, regulate, normalize and construct understandings of the physical body and the virtuous bio-citizen" (p. 838). It is our assertion that biopedagogies are entrenched in the processes of professional socialization that unfold in the pedagogical spaces of post-secondary health professions education and training.

The remainder of this chapter unfolds in three parts. First, we briefly review biopedagogies, and related concepts. Second, we explore the interface of biopedagogies and professional socialization to theorize how fat oppression is deployed in the pedagogical spaces of dietetics education. Our discussion of biopedagogies and professional socialization is accompanied by illustra-tive excerpts from interviews conducted as part of Meredith's master's thesis research, which was supervised by Jennifer. The interviews were conducted in late 2018 and early 2019 with students who were enrolled in either an undergraduate or graduate dietetics training program in Canada and who self-identified as fat, higher weight, "overweight," "obese," or otherwise identified as being in a larger body. Finally, we briefly discuss implications of this work to dietetics and health professions education and propose Rice's (2015) notion of body-becoming pedagogies as an alternative to biopedagogies, before offering concluding remarks.

Biopower and biopedagogies

Foucault originally theorized biopower in contrast to sovereign power (Foucault, 1978). Sovereign power is explicit, exercised through institutions, such as the penal system, and induces self-regulation among individuals through threat of potential punitive consequences of not doing so, such as being imprisoned or fined if one breaks a law. In contrast, biopower is the regulation of members of a population through the covert control of their bodies (Halse, 2009). As Harwood (2009) notes, "it is a power that appears life conserving, yet functions to *fortify populations* in the name of modern state power, commanding practices in the name of life (and whether these are indeed life enhancing is open to debate)" (p. 16–17).

Biopower has been further elaborated through a related concept, disciplinary power. Evans and Rich (2011) define disciplinary power as a form of power by which people

> are ascribed responsibility for regulating and looking after themselves, though often according to criteria over which they have very little say or control while, at the same time, being more or less relentlessly monitored in their capacity to do so. (pp. 364–365)

Disciplinary power is enacted as individuals self-monitor and internalize ideas and practices in line with governing norms that shape the limits of decency, respectability, and even what is possible. By aligning thoughts and behaviors with governing norms, individuals present themselves as good (read conscientious, responsible, moral) citizens. For example, "watching what one eats" to conform to dominant ideas of health is reflective of disciplinary power. The consequences for individuals who fail to conform are not fines and imprisonment as with sovereign power but comprise social sanctions and internalized shame.

For Phillips and Nava (2011), biopower and disciplinary power are symbiotic, but operate at different levels. Phillips and Nava theorize biopower as control exerted over populations, while disciplinary power is exercised at the level of individuals. To illustrate, Phillips and Nava (2011) problematize conceptualizations of the "good" Latino/a teacher who, through certain behavioral practices (i.e., disciplinary power) enacts their role in "passing and enforcing educational policies whose aim is to influence statistical norms of the population" (i.e., biopower, p. 4). We draw on, and expand, Phillips and Nava's two-tiered conceptualization of bio- and disciplinary power to make sense of the ways that fat oppression is perpetuated through the biopedagogies of professional socialization via the structures and norms of dietetics' pedagogical milieu (i.e., biopower) and fat dietetics students' agentive internalization, but more specifically corporealization of fat oppression in service of an embodied professional dietetics identity (i.e., disciplinary power).

Biopedagogies is a concept that draws heavily on Foucault's work. Recall that Wright and Halse (2014) describe biopedagogies as "the values and practices that are disseminated through informal education (e.g., media and Internet) as well as formal education (e.g., school) which work to instruct, regulate, normalize and construct understandings of the physical body and the virtuous bio-citizen" (p. 838). In the biopedagogical context of schools, "obese" children and children at risk of "obesity," which seemingly includes all children, are targets of health and education programs and policies that call upon children to manage their weight (Evans & Rich, 2011). Wright (2009) notes that some biopedagogies make explicit attempts to change behaviors, such as public health campaigns, while others present a more subtle nudge to influence individual behavior, such as the way that fat people are portrayed on television or in the media.

Rail (2012) has proposed the "Obesity Clinic" to theorize the diffuse and insidious ways that "anti-obesity" discourse entreats disciplinary relationships among individuals and between individuals and their bodies. For Rail, the "obesity clinic" is a clinic without borders. It is a biopedagogical system that functions by inviting specific types of behaviors by appealing to individuals' desire for risk aversion, responsibility, and to be seen as a "good biocitizen," a conscientious and moral individual that does the right things through self-surveillance and monitoring (Rail, 2012). Rail and Jette (2015) identify those who reject the lessons of biopedagogies as "bio-Others," and problematize the "rescue missions" that have been undertaken to save them, such as those led by various health professionals through their day-to-day practice and through public health campaigns (p. 328). In Rail and Jette's (2015) theorization of biopedagogies, fat people are among the abject caste of bio-Others. But what of those who are both the object and subject of biopedagogies, namely health professions' students? How might biopedagogies elucidate the process of becoming professional (i.e., professional socialization), which involves a repositioning of health professions students from an object position to one that is both object and subject? What of fat dietetics students who are marked as "bio-Others" and who are authorized to undertake "rescue missions" (Rail & Jette, 2015)? How are biopedagogies deployed in health professions education to construct, not the "virtuous bio-citizen" as in Wright and Halse's (2014) terms, but the virtuous health professional?

Expanding biopedagogies: Fat oppression in dietetics education

In this section we elucidate responses to questions, such as those posed above, that emerge at the interface of biopedagogies and professional socialization. In line with Phillips and Nava's (2011) two-tiered framework, we assert that biopedagogies interface with professional socialization at two levels: structural biopedagogies of dietetics education that operate at the collective or population level and comprise the explicit and implicit lessons about dietetics knowledge, skill, behaviors, comportment, attitudes, and values; and internalized biopedagogies that, through behaviors and other practices, are employed by dietetics students to demonstrate their emerging expertise and dietetics identity by quite literally fitting their cognitive, affective, and corporeal selves to the norms of the profession.

Structural and internalized biopedagogies operate symbiotically to give rise to a broader biopedagogical environment of fat oppression in which dietetics students learn what it means to be a dietitian. Course assignments provide a particularly illustrative example of the symbiosis of structural and internalized biopedagogies that are fundamental to professional socialization. Course assignments are an important means by which dietetics students are trained in the knowledge and skills of dietetics practice, but also by which they are inculcated in and enact via their own bodies the professions' norms, values, and judgements about body weight. Anthropometric and dietary data, such as height, weight, waist circumference, skin-fold thicknesses, and caloric intake are part of dietitians' routine assessments of clients' nutrition status. As such, dietetics students must demonstrate their ability to collect, interpret, and apply anthropometric and dietary intake data. Students are regularly expected to demonstrate such knowledge and skill through self- or peer-assessment assignments whereby students collect anthropometric and dietary data using themselves or fellow students, sometimes in front of faculty and peers. Conducting self- and peer-assessments intercedes upon students' bodies and bodily practices to draw intimate connections between the knowledge and skills they must acquire to validate their professional competence, but also their embodied submission to that knowledge and its implicit messages—managing one's weight is the result of and evidence that one comprehends and is adhering to dietetics knowledge. It is by drawing these intimate connections between biopower and disciplinary power that biopedagogies direct professional socialization and render the student as a "becoming professional." One dietetics student participant described her experience with a self-assessment assignment and therein highlights the highly gendered intersections of biopedagogies and professional socialization:

> There were different assessment techniques that we had to do and we were doing them all in front of each other, and one of them was everybody was getting weighed in front of everybody, and seeing the people cry, and it was just like…That impacts you in certain ways, like I understand it gives you a perspective of what a patient or client may feel if they have to do that in front of you as well, but this is also a highly competitive group of women all around each other, and it's just, that did not feel okay.

For health professions students, including dietetics students, demonstrating competence, such as by completing self- and peer-assessments, is as much about acquiring knowledge and skills, as it is about corporealizing those lessons.

Structural biopedagogies

Course assignments, interactions with faculty and peers, physical spaces, and the culture of competition associated with internship selection, are some of the important biopedagogical sites that impart explicit and implicit messages about what it means to be a dietetics student and an emerging professional. The physical space of dietetics education is an important biopedagogical site that disciplines the fat dietetics student body during professional socialization. Physical spaces within the education environment act to impart lessons that fat dietetics students' bodies do not fit, and thus require intervention, such as by professional expertise. Physical space as biopedagogy is not unique to health professions education. Brown (2018), Hetrick and Attig (2009), Royce (2016), and Stevens (2018) characterize educational, and public spaces more broadly, as biopedagogical in accommodating, and thereby normalizing, a narrow range of bodies. These authors' work explores the constraining nature of classroom desks, chairs, campus dining halls, and other campus spaces as examples of the biopedagogical function of physical space. Participants in Meredith's research also highlighted the physical constraints imposed on them by desks and chairs. One participant's description of the bathroom stalls at her university illuminates the role of physical space as biopedagogies as it exists outside of the classroom:

> But so far, everything else I've seen, um, for example, the, some bathroom stalls are of smaller size, I guess they're based on older makes, but the newer ones are bigger size, so that maybe someone who is larger than me should try to use some of the washrooms, the older washrooms, they would probably have an issue getting into it. Not per se getting into it, but moving, shuffling around, in it.

In this participant's experience, using the bathroom requires that one either find a stall that fits their body, or finds a way to "shuffle around" in it that accommodates their size. Both options imply the need for the student to make their bodies fit. What is unique about physical space as biopedagogies in the environments of health profession education is that the achievement is not only the discipline of fat bodies, but the concomitant production of professional identity and the reification of expert knowledge.

Interactions with faculty and student peers are another site where biopedagogies instill fat oppression within the processes of professional socialization. These interactions are often rife with judgement and discrimination, which further reinforces the notion that people in larger bodies cannot be effective dietitians. As one participant put it, fat dietetics students are often "being judged for the future of the profession on a different level"—as in, their body is on display as a sign or indication of their expertise, and if they are fat, it sends a negative message about not only them, but also the profession as a whole. Messages of judgement are often sent directly within dietetics education, but also often enforced by judgement that students receive from their broader social environment. These experiences of judgement are often tied up in what people expect dietitians to look like, and when dietetics students/dietitians do not meet those expectations, they often experience judgement. One participant described her experiences of judgment within dietetics in this way:

> Yeah, because there were, I would hear girls talking about how other girls were fat and to me, they looked not that different from the girls who were calling them fat, um, and they all looked perfect to me, so I was like, oh my god, what must they think of me? So it was just, there was a more open dialogue about being judgmental and negative when I was in my undergrad dietetics.

These experiences of judgement impact students, but also play a role in the weight bias that is often exhibited by dietitians toward people in larger bodies, as this student further highlighted:

> Well it's just the thing, if you can't talk to your classmates in a way that respects different bodies, how are you going to talk to a patient or a client

face to face who's in a much larger body, telling you about, you know, their eating binges or what have you.

This is important, as biopedagogies are not just built into the direct educational structure but also into the social structure within which dietetics students exist.

Finally, the culture of competition related to the internship application and selection process is an important biopedagogical site whereby explicit pronouncements are made about who has successfully demonstrated their acquisition of dietetics identity and who has not. One participant described the impact on internship competition in this way:

> Oh, [internship] breeds competitiveness, because you can, you know, no part of you was safe, people would attack your every action and kind of talk amongst themselves, that was a huge reason why I really couldn't get involved [in extracurricular activities], because I didn't want the way I looked to be personally attacked, more than I felt like it already was with like the looks and the comments.

This participant's insight highlights the ways that internship competition fuels disciplinary power, namely through self- and peer-surveillance. Brady and colleagues (2012, 2013) describe the internship candidate selection process as being guided by what they call "the fit…a vague constellation of attributes other than a candidate's determinable qualifications such as grade point average, work and volunteer experience, or education" which leaves the selection process open to "discrimination based on sex, race, body size, sexuality and so on" (2013, p. 7). Here, "the fit" takes on a double meaning to denote both the personal (i.e., attitudes, values, demeanor) and physical (i.e., thin) qualities that align with professional knowledge, skill, and identity.

Internalized biopedagogies

In the context of dietetics education, internalized biopedagogies encompass the ways in which dietetics students internalize, but also notably corporealize, fat oppression as they come to learn and adopt what it means to think, do, say, and look like a dietitian. Hence, for dietetics students, internalized biopedagogies are fundamental to being and becoming (a) professional, and include the behavioral enactments of dietetics identity, but also the embodied execution of dietetics knowledge and ways of knowing, which is evidenced by being thin, but not too thin.

The behavioral enactments of dietetics identity promulgated at the interface of biopedagogies and professional socialization include various practices through which students incorporated and performed what it means to be professional and to be a dietitian. To illustrate, one participant described the pressure she felt to bring a "leafy green salad" rather than a "potato salad with mayo" to a class potluck, and then added "God forbid you bring a cupcake for dessert." Another participant similarly explained,

> ...one of the reasons I still have a pretty good body image overall is because I still do have that perception that I consider myself to be a healthy person, um, or just being able to say that I can still move, I can still run, I can still do all these different things, um, and the fact that I did that as I was gaining the weight too, um, was, like it definitely contributed to just like maintaining that positive perspective.

The perceived need by participants, all of whom described their bodies as being larger than a desirable or "normal" weight range, to offset or compensate for their status as a bio-Other within their pedagogical environments, which are devised to beget (thin) dietitians, highlights the intersection of biopedagogies and professional socialization. Enacting disciplinary power by performing behaviors in line with dietetics' identity animates dietetics knowledge and professional authority while demonstrating students' submission to the professional socialization process, which participants highlighted as being a particularly important fat oppressive biopower.

The behaviors performed by students also reflected classed, gendered, and racialized notions of healthy eating. The food, meal, and eating practices performed by students typified what is considered healthy by dominant, Eurocentric, White culture in North America, and what is perpetuated by tools such as the Canada's Food Guide (Aiken, 2018; Beagan & Chapman, 2012; Health Canada, 2019). For example, students noted that foods like salmon, broccoli, overnight oats, and quinoa hold particular value and caché as healthy foods among their peers. As one participant noted: "I feel ashamed that I, when I take a sandwich for lunch, or if I decide to order pizza or something, and you know, it's like, when the girl beside me is eating her fancy little quinoa and chickpea and whatever else." Conversely, foods like pizza, Cheez Whiz, potato chips, and Gatorade elicited disgust, judgement, and mockery. The stigma students associated with Cheez Whiz, potato chips, and Gatorade, reflect the status of these foods beyond judgements of health, to their association with marginalized racial, class, and colonial identities. In an open letter to "bougie white people," Carino (2018) elucidates "spam stigma" as being rooted in racism, classism, and colonial histories that are perpetuated by dominant, and we would add biopedagogical, discourse of healthy eating. Like spam stigma, biopedagogical discourse of healthy eating in the dietetics educational environment does not simply ignore the social, economic, cultural, or historical meanings of food, but actively diminishes the relevance of those meanings to why and what people eat, silences the global origins of foods and the sometimes-diasporic people who produce and eat them, and ultimately reasserts White supremacy. In other words, the biopedagogical environment of dietetics education reifies what we call "values-added foods." The term value-added is often used to label foods that have higher market value, but lower cultural value, because of their post-production processing (i.e., processed foods). We propose the term "values-added foods" as an additional conceptual tool that may describe the way that foods (i.e., salmon, quinoa) serve as synecdoche of the wider biopedagogical discourse that assigns higher moral and cultural value to certain foods and the people who eat them.

The biopedagogical context of dietetics also comprises the predominantly White, female, middle-class students and faculty (Dietitians of Canada, 2011). Biopedagogies are not only shaped by assignments, such as anthropometric laboratories or discussions about "obesity." Rather, biopedagogies are also shaped by class, race, and gender interactions within and outside of the dietetics classroom. As an example, one participant who was an international student from China described the judgement that she experiences from friends and family, regarding her body size. For this student, the experience of being a racialized, and international, student adds an additional layer of complexity to her identity as an emerging dietitian, and to her interactions with peers and the physical spaces of dietetics education. It is important to consider how various axes of power interact and interconnect within dietetics spaces. Exploring how intersecting racial, gendered, and classed oppression bear on the biopedagogical environments of dietetics education is an important area for future research.

In addition to the behavioral enactments theorized by Phillips and Nava's (2011) conceptualization of disciplinary power, the corporealization of biopedagogies is particularly salient in the context of dietetics education and professional socialization. Several participants commented on the importance of their bodies as proof of their professional identity and acumen, or lack thereof. One participant explained:

> Somehow I just cannot relay confidence in doing those things, because you know, you don't have a good body figure yourself, how can you teach others to be healthy and maintain a healthy weight?

Working on the body corporealizes dietetics knowledge, animates professional authority, and stands as evidence of students' submission to the professional socialization process.

To make sense of the ways in which biopower and disciplinary power operate symbiotically and concomitantly with professional socialization, we propose another conceptual tool, the bio-operative, to theorize the intersections of biopedagogies, professional socialization, and the roles of health professionals in perpetuating fat oppression. Bio-operatives comprise those who are the target of biopedagogies, but because of their professional status and role, are also authorized to act in service of expanding the reach of biopower and translating its purpose to the techne of disciplinary power. Hence, bio-operatives are both the object and subject, or target and conduit, of biopedagogies. Theorizing the ontology of bio-operatives is key to expanding biopedagogies as a theoretical framework, including how bio-operatives come to be positioned as such, namely through health professional education and training.

Conclusion and ways forward

Biopedagogies are highly intertwined with professional socialization and, together, shape dietetics education, and likely that of other health professions. Structural biopedagogies immerse students in a biopedagogized learning environment that is then internalized, and importantly corporealized, through the processes of professional socialization whereby students adopt the values, attitudes, behaviors, and embodiment of what it means to be a dietitian. It is at the interface of biopedagogies and professional socialization that students are constituted as bio-operatives—individuals that are both disciplined via biopedagogies, but are also authorized to discipline the bodies of others as health professionals. These biopedagogies shape and constrain the professionalization of dietetics students and constrict the ways in which we think of dietetics professionals. This has implications for the wellbeing of dietetics students and professionals, and also for the profession as a whole, when we limit the profession to being about weight management and the management of unruly bodies.

How might dietetics and other health professions education move beyond the biopedagogical context of professional socialization? In answer to this question, we look to Rice's (2015) emerging concept of "body-becoming pedagogies" (p. 387). Rice posits that body-becoming pedagogies "ask us to question mechanistic models and moralistic biopedagogies, to let go of normative notions about able bodies, and to consider how our ways of knowing bodies might influence what they can be" (p. 392). Body-becoming pedagogies prompts questions about how health professions education might "create the conditions that will enable [students] to imagine other possibilities for their bodies" beyond difference and "abjectness," to "make space for more ethical responses to size differences" (Rice, 2015, p. 392). Rice asserts that body-becoming pedagogies counter proscriptive, (fat) oppressive pedagogical approaches by enabling individuals to tell the story of their bodies, but also hold space for the "stories that their bodies tell about them" (p. 392). That is, counter to the science-focused, positivist, biomedical paradigm that pervades health professions education, body-becoming pedagogies invite health professions educators to explore cultural, social, physical, and other forces that shape the possibilities of what bodies are and what they can become (Rice, 2015). Incorporating these pedagogies into dietetics education and training would require dietetics educators to do deep work about the stories they tell about their own unruly bodies, and those of their students and patients. How do we shift the stories we tell about bodies away from health imagined through biomedicine in health professions education like dietetics? Exploring these questions presents vast possibilities that can and should be explored if dietetics educators are to begin to redress the repercussions of biopedagogized professional socialization that are presented in this chapter through the voices of the participants in Meredith's master's thesis research.

This work is the first to theorize the interface of biopedagogies and professional socialization. There is copious opportunity to develop this work, which was not possible here given space constraints. Specifically, future writing should further explore the gendered, classed, and racialized aspects of biopedagogized professional socialization, to expand on what is briefly elaborated here. It is important to continue reflecting on how biopedagogies shape the professional socialization of dietetics students, and how these pedagogies shape the profession and the practice of dietetics.

References

Aiken, K. (2018, August 29). "White people food" is creating an unattainable picture of health. *Huffington Post*. https://www.huffingtonpost.ca/entry/white-people-food_n_5b75c270e4b0df9b093dadbb?guccounter=1

Aphramor, L., & Gingras, J. (2009). That remains to be said: Disappeared feminist discourses of fat in dietetic theory and practice. In E. Rothblum, & S. Solovay (Eds.), *The fat studies reader* (pp. 97–105). NYU Press.

Beagan, B., & Chapman, G. (2012). Meanings of food, eating and health among African Nova Scotians: "Certain things aren't meant for Black folk". *Ethnicity & Health, 17*(5), 513–529. https://doi.org/10.1080/13557858.2012.661844

Brady, J. (2018). Toward a critical, feminist sociology of expertise. *Journal of Professions and Organization, 5*, 123–138. https://doi.org/10.1093/jpo/joy004

Brady., J., Hoang, A., Siswanto, O., Riesel, J., & Gingras, J. (2013). Voices of distress: The emotional peril of not attaining a dietetic internship in Ontario. *Journal of Critical Dietetics, 1*(3), 6–14. ISSN: 1923–1237.

Brady, J., Hoang, A., Tzianetas, R., Buccino, J., Glynn, K., & Gingras, J. (2012). Unsuccessful dietetic internship applicants: A descriptive survey. *Canadian Journal of Dietetic Practice and Research, 73*(2), e248–e252.

Brown, H. A. (2018). "There's always stomach on the table and then I gotta write!" Physical space and learning in fat college women. *Fat Studies, 7*(1), 11–20. https://doi.org/10.1080/21604851.2017.1360665.

Carino, J. (2018). *Spam stigma: An open letter to White people*. https://www.vidaweb.org/spam-stigma-an-open-letter-to-white-people/

Dietitians of Canada. (2011). *The dietitian workforce in Canada: Meta-analysis report*. https://www.dietitians.ca/Downloads/Public/Workforce-Meta-Analysis-Report-English-pdf.aspx

Evans, J., & Rich, E. (2011). Body policies and body pedagogies: Every child matters in totally pedagogised schools? *Journal of Education Policy, 26*(3), 361–379. https://doi.org/10.1080/02680939.2010.500399

Foucault, M. (1978). *The history of sexuality. Volume 1: An introduction* (R. Hurley, Trans.). Pantheon Books.

Fraser, K., & Brady, J. (2018). Exploring social justice advocacy in dietetic education: A content analysis. *Canadian Journal of Dietetic Practice and Research, 80*(1), 2–7. https://doi.org/10.3148/cjdpr-2018-027.

Gingras, J., & Brady, J. (2010). Relational consequences of dietitians' feeding bodily difference. *Radical Psychology, 8*(1), 1–18.

Goldenberg, D., & Iwasiw, C. (1993). Professional socialization of nursing students as an outcome of a senior clinical preceptorship experience. *Nurse Education Today, 13*(1), 3–5.

Halse, C. (2009). Bio-citizenship: Virtue discourses and the birth of the bio-citizen. In J. Wright & V. Harwood (Eds.), *Biopolitics and the "obesity epidemic": Governing bodies* (pp. 45–59). Routledge.

Harwood, V. (2009). Theorizing biopedagogies. In J. Wright & V. Harwood (Eds.), *Biopolitics and the "obesity epidemic": Governing bodies* (pp. 15–30). Routledge.

Health Canada. (2019). *Canada's food guide.* https://food-guide.canada.ca/en/

Hetrick, A., & Attig, D. (2009). Sitting pretty: Fat bodies, classroom desks, and academic excess. In E. Rothblum, & S. Solovay (Eds.), *The fat studies reader* (pp. 197–204). New York University Press.

International Confederation of Dietetic Associations. (2014). *International standards.* https://www.internationaldietetics.org/International-Standards.aspx

Lordly, D., & MacLellan, D. (2012). Dietetic students' identity and professional socialization in preparation for practice. *Canadian Journal of Dietetic Practice and Research, 73*(1), 7. https://doi.org/10.3148/73.1.2012.7

MacLellan, D., Lordly, D., & Gingras, J. (2011). Professional socialization in dietetics: A review of the literature. *Canadian Journal of Dietetic Practice and Research, 72*(1), 37–42. https://doi.org/10.3148/72.1.2011.37

Phillips, D. K., & Nava, R. C. (2011). Biopower, disciplinary power, and the production of the "good Latino/a teacher." *Discourse: Studies in the Cultural Politics of Education, 32*(1), 71–83. https://doi.org/10.1080/01596306.2011.537074

Rail, G. (2012). The birth of the obesity clinic: Confessions of the flesh, biopedagogies, and physical culture. *Sociology of Sport Journal, 29*(2), 227–253.

Rail, G., & Jette, S. (2015). Reflections on biopedagogies and/of public health: On bio-others, rescue missions, and social justice. *Cultural Studies Critical Methodologies, 15*(5), 327–336. https://doi.org/10.1177/15327086.1561.1703

Rice, C. (2015). Rethinking fat: From bio- to body-becoming pedagogies. *Cultural Studies Critical Methodologies, 15*(5), 387–397. https://doi.org/10.1177/15327086.1561.1720

Rochefort, J. E., Senchuk, A., Brady, J., & Gingras, J. (2016). Spoon fed: Learning about "obesity" in dietetics. In J. Ellison, D. McPhail, & W. Mitchinson (Eds.), *Obesity in Canada: Critical perspectives* (pp. 148–174). University of Toronto Press.

Royce, T. (2016). Fat invisibility, fat hate: Towards a progressive pedagogy of size. In E. Cameron & C. Russell (Eds.), *The fat pedagogy reader: Challenging weight-based oppression through critical education* (pp. 21–30). Peter Lang.

Ruhl, J., & Lordly, D. (2017). The nature of competition in dietetics education: A narrative review. *Canadian Journal of Dietetic Practice and Research, 78*(3), 129–136. https://doi.org/10.3148/cjdpr-2017-004

Schaeffer, J. (2014, May). Dietitians and their weight struggles. *Today's Dietitian, 16*, 32. http://www.todaysdietitian.com/newarchives/050114p32.shtml

Siswanto, O., Brady, J., & Gingras, J. (2015). Successfully attaining a dietetic internship position in Ontario on the first attempt: A descriptive study. *Canadian Journal of Dietetic Practice and Research, 76*(1), 27–32. https://doi.org/10.3148/cjdpr-214-034

Stevens, C. (2018). Fat on campus: Fat college students and hyper(in)visible stigma. *Sociological Focus, 51*(2), 130–149. https://doi.org/10.1080/00380237.2017.1368839

Wright, J. (2009). Biopower, biopedagogies, and the obesity epidemic. In J. Wright & V. Harwood(Eds.), *Biopolitics and the "obesity epidemic": Governing bodies* (pp. 1–14). Routledge.

Wright, J., & Halse, C. (2014). The healthy child citizen: Biopedagogies and web-based health promotion. *British Journal of Sociology of Education, 35*(6), 837–855. https://doi.org/10.1080/01425692.2013.800446

6 A textbook case of bias

Virginia Dicken-Gracen

I discovered my love of teaching in the first grade. I would come home from school each day eager to teach my younger sister all I had learned. I felt that same sense of excitement when I landed my first tutoring gig in high school. And the rush returned when I was offered my first adjunct faculty position at a community college. This was what I had been waiting for, my entire reason for going to graduate school—to have classes of my own where I could develop lessons and share interesting ideas with students! My orientation to the position consisted of a chat with my new supervisor followed by a tour of the building and classrooms. At the end of the tour, I was handed a copy of the textbook used for all Introduction to Psychology classes on this campus. I had classrooms. I had a textbook. I felt incredible.

That night, I stayed up late mapping out possible syllabi for the upcoming semester. I started flipping through the book, imagining which in-class activities and demonstrations I could use to further explore each of the major concepts. And then I reached page 329.

"The World Health Organization has used the term globesity to refer to the worldwide problem of 'obesity,'" a set of large red text in the margins informed readers. Below it was a cartoon of a fat man wearing a poorly fitted shirt and pants that left his belly hanging exposed over the waistband. "I've got a complaint," he was saying as he handed a computer to a thin man in a suit behind a counter. "This laptop doesn't fit my lap!" (King, 2013).

My daydreams of what it would be like to teach my own classes shifted. Instead of picturing myself walking around a room, engaging learners in an interesting discussion about research methods, neurotransmitters, or adolescent development, I saw myself standing in front of a group of students with textbooks open to that page, seeing this comic mocking people with bodies that looked like mine. What else would they be told about me in this book? I flipped to the index to look for any other mentions of body size.

- "'Overweight' and 'obesity' are global health problems. Why people overeat to the point of 'obesity' is a motivational puzzle because it involves eating when one is not in need of nutrition" (p. 329).
- "'Overweight' and 'obesity' are second only to smoking in terms of controllable causes of death. Controllable means that these unhealthy conditions

DOI: 10.4324/9781003057000-7

of body composition can be influenced by behavior, specifically by eating patterns and physical activity levels" (p. 379).

- "Looking at the data cross-sectionally, the researchers found that neuroticism and extraversion were positively related to body weight. In contrast, conscientiousness was negatively related to body weight. These relationships were most strongly explained by impulsivity, a trait that involves acting without planning" (p. 379).

The final chapter of the textbook focused on health psychology and included an entire section conflating "obesity" with overeating and sedentariness, ironically citing Steven Blair's 1989 study of mortality trends while failing to mention that Blair's work found physical fitness is a much better predictor of mortality than body mass index (King, 2013).

Having studied size-inclusive approaches to health for several years, I recognized the problems with what I was reading in this textbook. But what good would such knowledge do for my students? Fat instructors who try to counter anti-fat narratives can be seen as biased and self-serving (Escalera, 2009).

I decided I was done with course planning for the night.

Over the next few weeks, with commiseration and advice from friends and colleagues, I returned to my excitement about those classes and found ways to work with and around that textbook, some of which I will describe later in this chapter. The experience did not diminish my passion for teaching, but the memory has stayed with me over the years as I've gone on to develop other classes in health services and sciences. The textbooks I have encountered in my subsequent academic experiences have been far less overt in their anti-fat content. None have included images that explicitly mock fat bodies. But outright mocking is not the only way that textbooks send negative messages about fatness.

Many health-related textbooks only mention body size when listing "high BMI" as a controllable behavioral risk-factor for negative health and social outcomes, substituting "overweight/obesity" as shorthand for poor nutrition or sedentary lifestyles, and treating weight loss or prevention of weight gain as a desirable goal.

A quick review of the collection of books on my office shelves produces the following examples:

- A mind/body health textbook that lists "obesity" among chronic illnesses such as diabetes and cardiovascular disease and warns of its impact on the economy in terms of treatment costs and lost productivity.
- A nutrition textbook that encourages establishing healthy eating habits in childhood to prevent later weight gain in adulthood, warning that developing such habits is often too late after "obesity" has set in.
- A health systems textbook that provides estimates of the medical spending attributable to "overweight and obesity" and comparing these costs to those of smoking.
- A diversity and inclusion textbook that warns "obesity" leads to psychosocial problems and "overweight" children are at risk of lifelong health challenges and damaging social stigma.

Those who are unfamiliar with size-inclusive health theory and practice might not see any problem with these examples. After all, textbook authors summarize the conclusions of current research, and most cite their primary sources appropriately. What is missing in these summaries, however, is a critical examination of how anti-fat bias has impacted the original research they are citing. Simply telling students about the amount of money spent on the treatment of "obesity" fails to recognize the role of the lucrative weight-loss industry and its efforts to convince customers that weight is largely controllable through their plans. Simply telling students that healthy dietary habits established in childhood make later weight gain less likely fails to acknowledge the many fat people who eat in balanced ways and reap the benefits of this behavior despite gaining weight as they age. Simply telling students that medical spending attributed to high body weight rivals that attributed to smoking fails to distinguish between body size and behaviors and assumes fat people would have the same health needs and outcomes as thin people if they could only find a way to avoid being fat people. Simply telling students that the "epidemic" of fatness leads to psychosocial problems and stigma fails to point out that the roots of such issues are the prejudices of society, not children's large bodies (a particularly surprising omission for a textbook about diversity and inclusion).

Such anti-fat bias in textbooks has been studied for over 20 years. In a 1999 project examining over two dozen abnormal psychology textbooks, Esther Rothblum found that most excluded research on the risks and ineffectiveness of dieting and other weight loss strategies. "Obesity" was addressed in sections focused on unhealthy behaviors or addiction and was presented as a life-threatening condition caused by lack of motivation. In 2014, Laura Jennings found that a sample of high school health textbooks presented fatness as incompatible with health, reinforced stereotypes about fat people, and provided contradictory messages about healthy behaviors and weight. The photos in these books often excluded fat people or portrayed them as unhappy, uncomfortable, incompetent, or inactive (e.g., showing two fat people riding an escalator next to an empty stairway).

The authors of these books did not independently produce the weight bias found in their writing. The bias existed in the research studies and professional culture that informed their work and was simply reproduced in their summaries. As instructors, we know that textbooks reflect current understandings and attitudes in a professional field. The creators of these resources are our colleagues. They are drawing from a large body of literature and trying to summarize it in a way that will make sense for students encountering these ideas for the first time. They bring with them their own training backgrounds and assumptions, so it is unsurprising that sizeism, a major bias in our health-related fields, finds its way into our textbooks.

Students do not have the same benefit of understanding how textbooks are developed and what strengths and limitations they bring to learning. Students tend to view textbooks as authoritative sources of information (Shapiro, 2012). What future health care providers encounter in these readings can have a lasting influence on their professional beliefs and practices. Additionally, fat- health professions students have shared how discouraging it is to face an overwhelmingly anti-fat curriculum (Dillon, 2016; Lomax-Sawyers, 2017). Those of us who care about sizeism in health care owe it to our students and their future patients to pay close attention to how fatness is discussed and portrayed in the readings we assign.

There are several strategies an instructor might use for dealing with textbook bias. Which ones a person will adopt depends heavily on their level of power in the teaching setting. As a teaching assistant in graduate school, I had limited power when a course professor assigned our undergraduate students to read about the "childhood obesity epidemic" and tasked me with grading their reading reflections. I sent him an article critiquing the anti-fat framework, and he posted it online in an "additional resources" section of our school's course management system. I knew that few students would make use of these optional readings, but there was little more I could do. Most teaching situations afford a teacher greater control than I experienced in that position. Here are a few options for using what power we have as instructors.

Strategy 1: Choose inclusive textbooks

The most direct solution for addressing bias in textbooks is to select inclusive texts and avoid those with anti-fat messages. If you are free to choose texts for your classes, you may be able to get review copies of books from publishers and search for keywords in the index. If you can obtain an electronic copy of the text, you can quickly search the entire contents, so you may want to ask the publisher if this is an option. Past research on textbook representations of fatness has used the following list of keywords to identify potentially relevant content (McHugh & Kasardo, 2012): body weight/shape, body image, dieting, eating disorders, eating, fat, fat oppression, "obesity," "overweight," overeating, and weight.

Phrases that begin with these keywords (such as "obesity epidemic" and "weight loss") should also appear when conducting a search, but variants (such as "obese") may not. I recommend adding the following terms: body mass index/BMI, fitness, nutrition, "obese," size, and sizeism.

As with all areas of human diversity, staying abreast of current issues and maintaining close contact with activists and educators working for inclusion will help you keep your own list of keywords up-to-date, as the language of oppression and social justice changes over time.

There is no simple formula for determining what qualifies as an acceptably inclusive textbook. Some instructors may seek out books that explicitly address anti-fat biases in health science and health practice. Others may find a text acceptable if it simply omits any mention of body size. Such choices will depend largely on your teaching style, course objectives, and plans for using the textbook.

In addition to searching for keywords, take note of any images in the book. Textbooks written for undergraduate and graduate level education are less likely to include images than those used in primary and secondary school settings, but many do still use stock photos and illustrations. This is especially true of introductory books and books for classes focused on anatomy or specific clinical skills. Do the images in the book represent a wide variety of body types in terms of race, ability, sex, and size? Are images of fat bodies presented neutrally or positively? Be especially aware of stereotype-congruent images of fat people and "headless fatty" pictures in which fat people are only shown from the neck down or from behind (Cooper, 2007). Exposure to stigmatizing images may increase anti-fat attitudes, while exposure to positive images of diverse bodies may improve attitudes toward both self and others (Ogden et al., 2020; Puhl et al., 2013).

Strategy 2: Assign selected chapters or sections

Sometimes we are stuck with a textbook that contains anti-fat material, whether because it was chosen for us or because there is no acceptable substitute. One option in this situation is to assign specific chapters or sections of the textbook and skip over others. This is the strategy I adopted to get through those first community college courses I taught. A mentor reminded me that the textbook need not dictate the course structure, and I still had a great deal of agency to design a syllabus and lesson plans that aligned with my values and my understanding of current research. Over the following semesters, however, I learned there are some important considerations/limitations to this using approach.

First, some students will still encounter the omitted reading material. This became clear to me when students were making use of the book's table of contents and index pages to complete their final papers. Each semester, there was a handful of students who would cite sections of the textbook I had not assigned as required reading earlier in the semester, including the anti-fat content.

Second, the best way to use this approach seems to be omitting entire chapters rather than sections or subsections of a chapter. Students may not be familiar with textbook organizational hierarchies, so assigning "Sections 1–3 and 5–7 of Chapter 10" can be confusing. Assigning specific page ranges can work better, but it is still more confusing than including or omitting an entire chapter. Of course, omitting an entire chapter may cut other critical material which will then need to be covered in greater detail in-class or through supplemental readings.

Skipping over chapters and sections with egregious anti-fat content allowed me to teach those first classes with some sense of integrity for a few years, but given the limitations of this strategy, I do not recommend it if other options are available to you.

Strategy 3: Supplement with inclusive material

A more active approach to handling textbook bias is to assign supplemental material that counters or provides context for the anti-fat messages, offering a fuller perspective. For example, if the textbook only mentions "obesity" as a risk factor for diseases, you might assign supplemental readings about conditions for which high BMI is a protective factor. If the textbook includes weight-loss as a recommendation for improving health outcomes, you might assign supplemental readings about weight-neutral or "Health at Every Size (HAES™)" approaches to health promotion.

Take care that your supplemental materials are high-quality, credible, and comprehensible to students in health-related fields. A study of critical fat scholars found that many instructors employ a strategy of "layering," presenting new ideas cautiously to move students over time, helping them unlearn previous ways of thinking about fatness without overwhelming them with critical theory perspectives (Cameron, 2015). Some of us find value in challenging the biomedical focus that too often dominates discussions about fatness, but material employing the traditional tools of health sciences—statistics, epidemiology, clinical research, etc.—may be more helpful for presenting a counterpoint to textbook literature that uses those same tools. At the same time, there is no reason to avoid sharing stories that illustrate principles of inclusive health care. Narratives can be compelling, and many critical fat scholars find their students connect well with real people's experiences (Cameron, 2015).

Do not assume students will automatically understand the differences between what they have read in their textbook chapter and what they have read in the supplemental material. As mentioned previously, students often see their textbooks as authoritative resources, transcending the influence of human culture or bias (Shapiro, 2012). Science-based courses are less likely than humanities courses to emphasize theory and cultural critique, so some health science students may be uncomfortable with questioning the textbook or grappling with contradictory messages in their assigned readings. Additionally, if the textbook confirms their previously held beliefs about weight and health, the supplemental material may be dismissed or misread.

One way to help students understand and wrestle with the differences between their textbook reading and their supplemental reading is to discuss the weight-normative and weight-inclusive approaches to health with them beforehand (Tylka et al., 2014). This will provide students with language and a framework for categorizing the divergent perspectives they are about to encounter and, hopefully, engaging with them more deeply.

Strategy 4: Customize an open educational resources textbook

Supplemental readings are no longer the only option for curating texts. Entire textbooks can be customized for a course thanks to the growing availability of open educational resources (OER) or "open textbooks." These resources are constantly changing, so I recommend working with your institution's library staff to see what is available to you. OER are typically low-cost or free digital textbooks with licenses that are more flexible than traditional textbook copyrights. This means you may be able to remix and modify the material, removing or updating sections and adding additional content. This can be a great way to provide students with a low-cost resource customized for your particular class to reflect inclusive and current research about size diversity and health. Students who are assigned open textbooks report using the text and enjoying it more than those assigned traditional print textbooks, and their learning outcomes are often similar or better

(Cuttler, 2019; Hilton, 2016). Students also appreciate the financial savings, and economic concerns are an important consideration when creating size-inclusive learning environments, as fat people experience disproportionate levels of poverty and employment discrimination (Han et al., 2009; Rudolph et al., 2009).

Strategy 5: Collaborate to create

This final strategy complements the previous strategies: work with those who create textbooks and other course materials. Offer your own knowledge about size-inclusive health science and practice. Textbooks are updated regularly, and there is no reason to assume that the next edition must include the same anti-fat material as the current edition. I am happy to report that more recent versions of the textbook I was assigned to teach from years ago no longer include that comic mocking fat people or the section on fat people's personality traits. I take no credit for these changes, as I did not understand my own power to reach out to the publisher or author at that point in my teaching career. We, as instructors, are part of a knowledge producing community. Whether we share size-inclusive resources with colleagues who are writing textbooks, serve as textbook reviewers, or work with others to develop new OER, we can play an active role in shaping which options are available for future classes.

A final note: There has been some push to move away from using textbooks in college courses. The price of textbooks has risen over 1,000% in the past 50 years (Popken, 2015). Instructors and students have more alternative resources at their disposal than ever before. Nevertheless, I foresee textbooks continuing to be important in health professions education. They provide organized summaries of our ever-expanding scientific knowledge. Most textbooks support student learning by highlighting key vocabulary terms, structuring complex information with charts and diagrams, and inviting students to assess their own understanding with self-check questions and chapter reviews. A good textbook can be invaluable.

But textbooks do not teach a course. Whether we teach online or face-to-face, instructors are responsible for bringing course content to life and guiding students as they make meaning of it. Finding (or creating) an inclusive and accurate set of readings for our students is unlikely to change their beliefs about fatness and fat people unless we prepare them for the reading assignments and provide them opportunities to discuss and apply what they have encountered in the text.

This became particularly apparent to me when my family was recently preparing to move to a new state. Like many academics, I decided a move was a good opportunity to clear out some of the resources I'd acquired over the course of my own education. While going through the books and boxes of materials, I came across a reading from my first semester of graduate school over 15 years ago. This reading discussed research showing the benefits of a non-weight-loss approach to health promotion for fat individuals. I was surprised to discover this in my sorting because I distinctly recalled my first exposure to such research came a year later as I was traveling to the annual American Public Health Association conference. I was a diligent student, so I am certain I did not skip the assignment that first semester. Somehow, though, it did not affect my understanding of fatness. In fact, the following semester I began planning a thesis on how people might be encouraged to make "healthy weight loss choices." While I do not remember the specifics of that first semester, I suspect one reason this reading did not leave an impression on me was that it was assigned in a research methods class. Our in-class discussions likely focused on the research design and analysis, not the topic of size-inclusive health promotion. An equally likely explanation for my lack of response to this reading is that I was personally invested in my own dreams of weight loss at the time.

The messages students encounter in our assigned class readings are always competing with the loud, living text of the world around them—television shows mocking fat bodies, peers discussing their diet plans, headlines about the "obesity epidemic," magazine and billboard images promoting the thin ideal, health care providers using weight as a proxy for health. As instructors, each of us must decide how much we can, should, and will do to counter those messages in our specific educational contexts. Assigning weight-neutral and size-inclusive readings avoids compounding these sizeist "public pedagogies." But to truly transform our students' understandings of body size and health, we must engage them in challenging conversations about their texts—both those we've assigned in class and those that surround them in their personal and professional worlds.

References

Cameron, E. (2015). Toward a fat pedagogy: A study of pedagogical approaches aimed at challenging obesity discourse in post-secondary education. *Fat Studies*, 4(1), 28–45. http://doi.org/10.1080/21604851.2015.979336

Cooper, C. (2007, January 7). *Headless fatties*. http://charlottecooper.net/fat/fat-writing/headless-fatties-01-07/

Cuttler, C. (2019). Students' use and perceptions of the relevance and quality of open textbooks compared to traditional textbooks in online and traditional classroom environments. *Psychology Learning & Teaching*, 18(1), 65–83. https://doi.org/10.1177/1475725718811300

Dillon, J. D. (*Host*). (2016, March 7). Love food podcast episode 008: I am a fat nutrition student. [Audio podcast.] https://juliedillonrd.com/love-food-podcast-episode-008-i-am-a-fat-nutrition-student/

Escalera, E. A. (2009). Stigma threat and the fat professor: Reducing student prejudice in the classroom. In E. Rothblum & S. Solovay (Eds.), *The fat studies reader* (p. 205–212). New York University Press.

Han, E., Norton, E. C., & Stearns, S. C. (2009). Weight and wages: Fat versus lean paychecks. *Health Economics*, 18, 535–548. https://doi.org/10.1002/hec.1386

Hilton, J. (2016). Open educational resources and college textbook choices: A review of research on efficacy and perceptions. *Educational Technology Research and Development*, 64, 573–590. https://doi.org/10.1007/s11423-016-9434-9

Jennings, L. (2014). Visual representation of fatness and health in high school health texts. *Fat Studies: An Interdisciplinary Journal of Body Weight and Society*, 3(1), 45–57. https://doi.org/10.1080/21604851.2013.784946

King, L. A. (2013). *Experience psychology* (2nd ed.). McGraw-Hill Education.

Lomax-Sawyers, I. (2017). On being a fat medical student, at the start of our metabolism module. *Journal of Paediatrics and Child Health*, 53(8), 733–734. https://doi.org/10.1111/jpc.13648

McHugh, M. C., & Kasardo, A. E. (2012). Anti-fat prejudice: The role of psychology in explication, education, and eradication. *Sex Roles*, 66(9–10), 617–627. https://doi.org/10.1007/s11199-011-0099-x

Ogden, J., Gosling, C., Hazelwood, M., & Atkins, E. (2020). Exposure to body diversity images as a buffer against the thin-ideal: An experimental study. *Psychology, Health & Medicine*, 1–14. https://doi.org/10.1080/13548506.2020.1734219

Popken, B. (2015). *College textbook prices have risen 1041 percent since 1977*. https://www.nbcnews.com/feature/freshman-year/college-textbook-prices-have-risen-812-percent-1978-n399926

Puhl, R. M., Luedicke, J., & Heuer, C. A. (2013). The stigmatizing effect of visual media portrayals of obese persons on public attitudes: Does race or gender matter? *Journal of Health Communication*, 18, 805–826. https://doi.org/10.1080/10810730.2012.757393

Rothblum, E. (1999). Contradictions and confounds in coverage of obesity: Psychology journals, textbooks, and the media. *Journal of Social Issues*, 55(2), 355–369. https://doi.org/10.1111/0022-4537.00120

Rudolph, C. W., Wells, C. L., Weller, M. D., & Baltes, B. B. (2009). A meta-analysis of empirical studies of weight-based bias in the workplace. *Journal of Vocational Behavior*, 74, 1–10. https://doi.org/10.1016/j.jvb.2008.09.008

Shapiro, A. R. (2012). Between training and popularization. Regulating science textbooks in secondary education. *Isis*, 103(1), 99–110. https://doi.org/10.1086/664981

Tylka, T. L., Annunziato, R. A., Burgard, D., Daníelsdóttir, S., Shuman, E., Davis, C., & Calogero, R. M. (2014). The weight-inclusive versus weight-normative approach to health: Evaluating the evidence for prioritizing well-being over weight loss. *Journal of Obesity*. https://doi.org/10.1155/2014/983495

7 Why would I want to come back?

Weight stigma and noncompliance

Nancy Ellis-Ordway

He said that everything that is wrong with me is my own fault, because of my life-style, that I brought the diabetes on myself! He said I was noncompliant! I'll show him noncompliant! I'm never going back to him again! I may never go to the doctor again at all!" Clarissa, a client, told me in a session.[i] Clarissa is on disability because of depression and has been seeing me for quite some time for counseling. We have talked about good nutrition and physical activity as aspects of self care, especially when she does not feel deserving of it. All of the improvements we have worked on have just been undone by her disapproving endocrinologist.

We choose careers in the health care professions because we want to help people live the healthiest, best quality lives possible. Whether we are doctors, nurses, physical therapists, social workers, dieticians, epidemiologists, counselors, schedulers, or other allied health professionals, we want everyone to have access to high-quality health care. If we are serious, we continue to look for ways to learn, grow and improve.

Medical care, however excellent, is ineffective if it is not utilized. The best recommendations in medical care and public health will only work if the people to whom they are directed follow through with them. How do we address non-compliance in our practices and our professions?

Background and literature review

Different terminology is used to describe this phenomenon, including compliance, persistence and adherence (Cramer et al., 2008) or even "patient disobedience" (Krot & Sousa, 2017, p. 79). Despite the different levels of disparagement implied in these terms, they all refer to a failure to follow directions regarding medication, behavior, or follow-up care.

Patient compliance influences both clinical and economic benefits for individuals and health care systems (Krot & Sousa, 2017). Noncompliance can result in incomplete treatment, delays in diagnosis, and missed opportunities for prevention. Patients are unlikely to receive full benefit of treatment (Eraker et al., 1984) if they do not adhere to instructions. Compliance has an impact on morbidity and mortality (Cramer et al., 2008).

Sometimes recommendations are misunderstood, forgotten, or ignored. Patients may not be able to understand the directions because of the way they

DOI: 10.4324/9781003057000-8

are given, or they may not be able to remember them later. Motivation is affected by the patient's perception of both the risk of the ailment and the benefits of the treatment. Side effects and costs also potentially interfere with compliance (Whitworth, 2017a).

Suggestions for improving compliance include such ideas as educating the patient, explaining goals more thoroughly, improving health literacy, asking about potential financial constraints, asking the patient to repeat back the instructions (Whitworth, 2017b) and improving social support (DiMatteo, 2004). Compliance improves when patients trust the benevolence, integrity, and honesty of their doctor (Krot & Sousa, 2017).

Effective communication is often listed as a modifiable factor to improve compliance (Zolnierek & DiMatteo, 2009), but rarely is weight stigma on the part of the medical professional considered as a possible influence. Weight stigma is a known cause for delayed or avoided medical care, but it is rarely addressed in an effective way.

Recommendations for addressing weight in health care are confusing, contradictory, and sometimes contentious. The United States Preventive Services Task Force guidelines recommend screening and behavioral interventions for those with a higher body mass index (BMI; Moyer & U. S.Preventive Services Task Force, 2012) but overlook the fact that higher weight is itself a stigmatized condition. Focusing on weight risks alienating and humiliating the very patients we are trying to help (Phelan et al., 2015). Meanwhile, there is no convincing evidence that these interventions result in either improved health or weight loss (Bacon & Aphramor, 2011; Bombak, 2014; Mann et al., 2007; Rothblum, 2018; Tylka et al., 2014).

The terms weight stigma, weight bias, and anti-fat bias all refer to the social rejection and/or devaluation based on having a body size that does not conform to social norms or expectations (Tomiyama et al., 2018). Weight stigma can be explicit and conscious or implicit and outside of awareness. While most health care practitioners will not deliberately set out to harm the people seeing them for care, implicit negative attitudes toward those in larger bodies have the potential to interfere in the relationship and negatively affect outcome.

Weight bias in health professions education

"The whole PowerPoint presentation was full of microaggressions; it was so shaming toward people in larger bodies. The emphasis was on dieting and restricting, it sounded dangerous, but I couldn't leave. And now it will be on the final!" Julie fought hard to recover from anorexia nervosa. She saw me for several years of follow-up treatment after her inpatient stay until she felt sufficiently recovered to stop therapy. A year later, she returned for support in dealing with the pressures of nursing school. She was unprepared for the weight stigma she would be exposed to in her training.

Weight bias in health care professionals and students is widely documented in the literature. In one study, 74% of medical students exhibited implicit weight bias and 67% indicated explicit bias (Phelan et al., 2014). Students in post-graduate training in a health discipline often observed weight stigma in their training (Puhl et al., 2014). Weight bias has been documented in dietetics students (Puhl et al., 2009) and physicians (Sabin et al., 2012). Anti-fat bias affects psychotherapists (Kinavey & Cool, 2019), nursing students (George et al., 2019) and physical therapists (Setchell et al., 2016). A commonly held stereotype among health care professionals is that heavier patients will be noncompliant because they are lazy or weak-willed (Phelan et al., 2015). When doctors believe that "obesity" is a disease which can be blamed on the patient, they convey that attitude to the patient (Eisenberg et al., 2019). Given the pervasiveness of weight bias among clinicians, it should not be surprising that people who fall into the categories of "overweight" and "obese" might want to avoid exposure to unpleasant encounters.

It is not unexpected to find weight bias among clinicians, given that the current widely accepted paradigm is "weight normative" (Tylka et al., 2014, p. 364), which is based on the disproven ideas that weight is under individual control and that weight loss results in improved health. Failure of weight loss attempts, which happens as much as 95% of the time, results in shame, guilt, body dissatisfaction, and health care avoidance (Mensinger et al., 2018; Tylka et al., 2014). Weight cycling, or losing and regaining more than once, is associated with a host of physical and mental consequences, such as metabolic changes (Neumark-Sztainer et al., 2006), increased cortisol levels (Bangalore et al., 2017), and reduced well-being, mental health and quality of life (O'Hara & Gregg, 2006). The widely accepted "weight normative" model considers that patients are harming their health by being fat, when in fact they are harming their health by weight cycling when they are trying to follow recommendations to make themselves smaller.

Weight stigma, in and of itself, is linked to many of the medical concerns that are blamed on excess weight. In one study, perceived weight discrimination explained 27% of dysregulation in metabolic markers (Daly et al., 2019). Internalized weight stigma is associated with disordered eating, low self-esteem, emotional dysregulation, lower levels of physical activity and poorer psychological well-being (Mensinger et al., 2018). Weight stigma also interferes with access to health care (Lee & Pausé, 2016).

Members of minority or marginalized groups are often less likely to access primary or preventative care due to concerns about poor treatment. Racial disparities in medicine are well documented among African Americans, Native Americans, and Latinos. This leads to higher levels of medical mistrust which then leads to lower levels of compliance with health recommendations (Armstrong et al., 2007; Frakt, 2020; Joszt, 2019; Kinlock et al., 2017; Williams, 2017). Similarly, biased attitudes toward gay, lesbian, or trans patients affect the likelihood of those individuals seeking medical attention (Tortelli, 2016). If heterosexual, cisgender, middle class, White women with health insurance report avoiding medical care due to weight stigma (Amy et al., 2006), how much more difficult is it for those with two or more marginalized identities to feel comfortable accessing medical care?

Weight stigma and compliance

The tension is visible in her posture. She wrings her hands, squeezing first one, then the other. "I know I need to go back on antidepressants, but that means I have to go to the doctor. I'm afraid of being lectured about my weight, that I won't be able to get a prescription unless I go on another diet." Emily is often unable to get out of bed to go to work because of her depression and anxiety. She is only seeing me because her family insisted. What reassurance can I offer her when I have heard so many stories like this?

Preventative screening is one of the most effective interventions in minimizing the effects of devastating diseases such as cancer, but they only work when they are utilized. For instance, "obesity" in women appears to be correlated with increased risk from gynecological cancers but higher weight women are less likely to obtain screening because of the way they have been treated, and expect to be treated at the doctor's office (Amy et al., 2006). Women who had been involved in more weight loss programs were more likely to avoid care (Daly et al., 2019).

Weight stigma from a doctor diminishes compliance (Hayward et al., 2020) and increases avoidance of preventative care (Sabin et al., 2012). Women in particular avoid or delay seeking health care because of fear of being fat-shamed or lectured about weight loss (Mensinger et al., 2018). Reasons for avoiding health care that are associated with weight stigma include: disrespectful treatment and negative attitudes on the part of staff, unsolicited recommendations for weight loss, embarrassment about being weighed, inadequately sized medical equipment (Puhl & Heuer, 2010), and previous poor treatment such as being berated about their weight (Drury & Louis, 2002).

A related issue is "doctor shopping." Having a consistent primary care physician improves continuity and quality of care. Negative interactions with health care providers, including nurses, clerks, and other personnel as well as doctors, prompt many patients to look for a new physician. Being shamed about body size or lectured about weight loss may impel a person to find a new provider. Weight bias contributes to increased doctor shopping in higher weight patients (Gudzune et al., 2013). Finding a physician's office that feels more comfortable is a better outcome than simply giving up on health care altogether, but perhaps doctor shopping could be minimized by focusing on making more offices welcoming to patients of size.

Leslie is a very thin, middle-aged woman who has finally found some relief from overwhelming anxiety and obsessional thinking since I talked her into trying a serotonin reuptake inhibitor. Her weight has drifted up very slightly as she has begun to take better care of herself. "The nurse practitioner won't refill my prescription unless I go back to see her! I can't let her see how fat I've gotten! She will yell at me!"

The language we use when we talk about both personal and public health often inadvertently reinforces weight stigma. Encouragement to "maintain a healthy weight" may sound kind but is vague enough to cause anxiety. How can patients know if they are getting it right? What is a "healthy weight?" Even slender individuals may believe that a "healthy weight" is "less than I weigh now."

It is important to recognize that weight stigma affects people of all sizes. When disparaging comments about large people go unchallenged, the message is clearly "Don't ever let yourself get fat like that!" Headlines about the threat of the

"Obesity Epidemic" reinforce the belief that gaining weight is the worst possible thing that can happen. Community-based interventions that emphasize weight loss as a goal support the belief that weight is controllable and everyone should just work harder to be thin.

One phrase that is particularly troublesome is "preventable deaths." While this term has a specific meaning in research and public health, it is sometimes used in the popular press. When it is used in connection with "obesity," it sounds like, "These deaths would have been prevented if people just got up off their lazy butts and lost weight!" Since articles identifying increased risk in higher weights usually then recommend more diligent medical screenings for those at risk (Wee et al., 2000), perhaps it would improve compliance if the phrasing did not involve blaming and shaming.

Recommendations for change

Public health

Weight stigma is also found in the field of public health. Interventions that focus on weight loss have a limited evidence base and they run the risk of further alienating the people they are designed to help. Fat shaming messages both encourage and condone discrimination. Educational programs should focus on stigma reduction rather than weight reduction. A weight-neutral public health agenda that includes a focus on improving access to a variety of foods, safe places to exercise and over-all quality of life for people of all sizes is a more promising strategy (Bombak, 2014).

Public health interventions should be evidence based and should focus on health and healthy behaviors rather than "obesity prevention." Using the terms "overweight" and "obesity" reinforces weight stigma and should be avoided. Compassion-centered programs to promote self-care, self-esteem, and body satisfaction are more likely to result in improved health behaviors than programs based on shaming and blaming. Educational interventions can promote respect for body size diversity even as they focus on improved understanding of the futility of weight loss attempts (Bacon & Aphramor, 2011).

Improving relationships in treatment settings

In medical practices, how do we improve compliance by increasing the number of our patients who want to come back to see us? How do we create safety for our patients of all sizes? How do we design an experience that helps them tell their stories? How do we craft a space that they want to return to? How do we send a clear message that all our patients are welcomed and valued in our setting? What needs to change about us, as medical professionals, that such a process is not only comfortable, but second nature?

A number of strategies to address weight stigma can enhance patient-provider relationships and thus improve compliance with recommendations. Training for practicing clinicians and students alike should include information about weight being determined by factors outside of individual control, and about the dismal outcomes of weight loss attempts. Education should include a component about the ethical issues, especially informed consent, involved in recommending an intervention that is likely to fail at the same time that it causes more problems. In addition, a zero-tolerance policy regarding comments or humor based on body size will challenge anti-fat bias in workplaces and schools (Phelan et al., 2015).

Make the space more welcoming by having larger gowns and blood pressure cuffs as well as wide chairs. Evaluate printed material, such as pamphlets, posters, and handouts for stigmatizing images and content. Consider the routine practices of the office that may communicate weight bias (Drury & Louis, 2002). While some medical conditions require frequent weight checks, avoidance of the scale is frequently listed as a reason to avoid or delay care. Many doctor's visits do not require weighing. If it is necessary to weigh a patient, do so with tact and sensitivity, and in a private space. No comment is required beyond "Thank you." If the patient prefers to get on the scale backwards to avoid the number (a common practice in the treatment of eating disorders), be respectful of that by not commenting about the number or whether it has gone up or down.

When talking with patients, ask about nutrition and physical activity levels before making recommendations. Focus on the behaviors of eating a wide variety of foods, especially fruits and vegetables, and maintaining a reasonable amount of physical activity. Avoid talk that emphasizes weight loss. If a patient asks for weight loss advice, explain the benefits of focusing on healthier behaviors instead. Avoid praising weight loss, as you may inadvertently be encouraging disordered eating behaviors. Remember that scolding a patient for weight gain increases the likelihood of never seeing that person again.

Consider drafting an office policy that includes all of these recommendations so that all of the staff understands the importance of compassionate, weight-neutral care. It might include specific instructions regarding when and how to weigh patients, guidelines for using larger equipment (such as blood pressure cuffs) and additional resources for learning about weight neutral approaches to treatment. A written policy makes clear that weight stigmatizing behaviors or attitudes are not acceptable.

The concept of trauma-informed care is a relatively recent and growing focus in training and clinical care. This framework recognizes that experiences of trauma can affect both health and utilization of health care (Dichter et al., 2018). Ideally, medical professionals can recognize and mitigate the needs of traumatized individuals; at a minimum, we should try to avoid exacerbating distress. It is vitally important to recognize weight stigma as contributing to trauma, especially when it is associated with health care.

Conclusion

Jennifer explains to me why she avoids doctors and describes a long list of experiences of being shamed at different weights. She discovered a psychiatrist who uses telemedicine to manage her prescriptions. "I wasn't scared because I knew they wouldn't weigh me!" She went on to say, "Now I'm thinking I also don't trust conventional doctors because they use more bias than actual science so how can you trust them with anything else?"

As clinicians, when we provide care to our patients and clients, we strive to do so in an atmosphere of a trusting, connected relationship. When our patients can feel confident in our honesty, benevolence, compassion, and caring, they will continue to see us and to follow our recommendations. The outcome is good medical care. And isn't that the goal?

References

Amy, N. K., Aalborg, A., Lyons, P., & Keranen, L. (2006). Barriers to routine gynecological cancer screening for White and African-American obese women. *International Journal of Obesity, 30*(1), 147–155. https://doi.org/10.1038/sj.ijo.0803105

Armstrong, K., Ravenell, K. L., McMurphy, S., & Putt, M. (2007). Racial/ethnic differences in physician distrust in the United States. *American Journal of Public Health, 97*(7), 1283–1289. https://doi.org/10.2105/AJPH.2005.080762

Bacon, L., & Aphramor, L. (2011). Weight science: Evaluating the evidence for a paradigm shift. *Nutrition Journal, 10*(1), 9. https://doi.org/10.1186/1475-2891-10-9

Bangalore, S., Fayyad, R., Laskey, R., DeMicco, D. A., Messerli, F. H., & Waters, D. D. (2017). Body-weight fluctuations and outcomes in coronary disease. *New England Journal of Medicine, 376*(14), 1332–1340. https://doi.org/10.1056/NEJMoa1606148

Bombak, A. (2014). Obesity, Health at Every Size, and public health policy. *American Journal of Public Health, 104*(2), e60–e67. https://doi.org/10.2105/AJPH.2013.301486

Cramer, J. A., Roy, A., Burrell, A., Fairchild, C. J., Fuldeore, M. J., Ollendorf, D. A., & Wong, P. K. (2008). Medication compliance and persistence: Terminology and definitions. *Value in Health: The Journal of the International Society for Pharmacoeconomics and Outcomes Research, 11*(1), 44–47. https://doi.org/10.1111/j.1524-4733.2007.00213.x

Daly, M., Sutin, A. R., & Robinson, E. (2019). Perceived weight discrimination mediates the prospective association between obesity and physiological dysregulation: Evidence from a population-based cohort. *Psychological Science, 30*(7), 1030–1039. https://doi.org/10.1177/0956797619849440

Dichter, M., Teitelman, A., Klusaritz, H., Maurer, D., Cronholm, P., & Doubeni, C. (2018). Trauma-informed care training in family medicine residency programs results from a CERA survey. *Family Medicine, 50*(8), 617–622. https://doi.org/10.22454/FamMed.2018.505481

DiMatteo, M. R. (2004). Social support and patient adherence to medical treatment: A meta-analysis. *Health Psychology, 23*(2), 207. https://doi.org/10.1037/0278-6133.23.2.207

Drury, C. A., & Louis, M. (2002). Exploring the association between body weight, stigma of obesity, and health care avoidance. *Journal of the American Academy of Nurse Practitioners, 14*(12), 554–561. https://doi.org/10.1111/j.1745-7599.2002.tb00089.x

Eisenberg, D., Noria, S., Grover, B., Goodpaster, K., & Rogers, A. M. (2019). ASMBS position statement on weight bias and stigma. *Surgery for Obesity and Related Diseases, 15*(6), 814–821. https://doi.org/10.1016/j.soard.2019.04.031

Eraker, S. A., Kirscht, J. P., & Becker, M. H. (1984). Understanding and improving patient compliance. *Annals of Internal Medicine, 100*(2), 258–268. https://doi.org/10.7326/0003-4819-100-2-258

Frakt, A. (2020). Race and medicine: The harm that comes from mistrust. *The New York Times TheUpshot: The New Health Care.* https://www.nytimes.com/2020/01/13/upshot/race-and-medicine-the-harm-that-comes-from-mistrust.html

George, T. P., DeCristofaro, C., & Murphy, P. F. (2019, September). Unconscious weight bias among nursing students: A descriptive study. *Healthcare, 7*(3), 106. https://doi.org/10.3390/healthcare7030106

Gudzune, K. A., Bleich, S. N., Richards, T. M., Weiner, J. P., Hodges, K., & Clark, J. M. (2013). Doctor shopping by overweight and obese patients is associated with increased healthcare utilization. *Obesity, 21*(7), 1328–1334. https://doi.org/10.1002/oby.20189

Hayward, L. E., Neang, S., Ma, S., & Vartanian, L. R. (2020). Discussing weight with patients with overweight: Supportive (not stigmatizing) conversations increase compliance intentions and health motivation. *Stigma and Health, 5*(1), 53. https://doi.org/10.1037/sah0000173

Joszt, L. (2019). *5 things about medical mistrust*. AJMC. https://www.ajmc.com/newsroom/5-things-about-medical-mistrust

Kinavey, H., & Cool, C. (2019). The broken lens: How anti-fat bias in psychotherapy is harming our clients and what to do about it. *Women & Therapy, 42*(1–2), 116–130. https://doi.org/10.1080/02703149.2018.1524070

Kinlock, B. L., Parker, L. J., Bowie, J. V., Howard, D. L., LaVeist, T. A., & Thorpe, R. J., Jr. (2017). High levels of medical mistrust are associated with low quality of life among Black and White men with prostate cancer. *Cancer Control: Journal of the Moffitt Cancer Center, 24*(1), 72–77. https://doi.org/10.1177/107327481702400112

Krot, K., & Sousa, J. P. (2017). Factors impacting on patient compliance with medical advice: Empirical study. *Engineering Management in Production and Services, 9*(2), 73–81. https://doi.org/10.1515/emj-2017-0016

Lee, J. A., & Pausé, C. J. (2016). Stigma in practice: Barriers to health for fat women. *Frontiers in Psychology, 7*, 2063. https://doi.org/10.3389/fpsyg.2016.02063

Mann, T., Tomiyama, A. J., Westling, E., Lew, A. M., Samuels, B., & Chatman, J. (2007). Medicare's search for effective obesity treatments: Diets are not the answer. *American Psychologist, 62*(3), 220–233. https://doi.org/10.1037/0003-066X.62.3.220

Mensinger, J. L., Tylka, T. L., & Calamari, M. E. (2018). Mechanisms underlying weight status and healthcare avoidance in women: A study of weight stigma, body-related shame and guilt, and healthcare stress. *Body Image, 25*, 139–147. https://doi.org/10.1016/j.bodyim.2018.03.001

Moyer, V. A., & United States Preventive Services Task Force. (2012). Screening for and management of obesity in adults: US preventive services task force recommendation statement. *Annals of Internal Medicine, 157*(5), 373–378. https://doi.org/10.7326/0003-4819-157-5-201209040-00475

Neumark-Sztainer, D., Wall, M., Guo, J., Story, M., Haines, J., & Eisenberg, M. (2006). Obesity, disordered eating, and eating disorders in a longitudinal study of adolescents: How do dieters fare 5 years later? *Journal of the American Dietetic Association, 106*(4), 559–568. https://doi.org/10.1016/j.jada.2006.01.003

O'Hara, L., & Gregg, J. (2006). The war on obesity: A social determinant of health. *Health Promotion Journal of Australia, 17*(3), 260–263. https://doi.org/10.1071/HE06260

Phelan, S. M., Burgess, D. J., Yeazel, M. W., Hellerstedt, W. L., Griffin, J. M., & van Ryn, M. (2015). Impact of weight bias and stigma on quality of care and outcomes for patients with obesity. *Obesity Reviews, 16*(4), 319–326. https://doi.org/10.1111/obr.12266

Phelan, S. M., Dovidio, J. F., Puhl, R. M., Burgess, D. J., Nelson, D. B., Yeazel, M. W., Hardeman, R., Perry, S., & Van Ryn, M. (2014). Implicit and explicit weight bias in a national sample of 4,732 medical students: The medical student CHANGES study. *Obesity, 22*(4), 1201–1208. https://doi.org/10.1002/oby.20687

Puhl, R. M., & Heuer, C. A. (2010). Obesity stigma: Important considerations for public health. *American Journal of Public Health, 100*(6), 1019–1028. https://ajph.aphapublications.org/doi/abs/10.2105/AJPH.2009.159491

Puhl, R. M., Luedicke, J., & Grilo, C. M. (2014). Obesity bias in training: Attitudes, beliefs, and observations among advanced trainees in professional health disciplines. *Obesity, 22*(4), 1008–1015. https://doi.org/10.1002/oby.20637

Puhl, R., Wharton, C., & Heuer, C. (2009). Weight bias among dietetics students: Implications for treatment practices. *Journal of the American Dietetic Association, 109*(3), 438–444. https://doi.org/10.1016/j.jada.2008.11.034

Rothblum, E. D. (2018). Slim chance for permanent weight loss. *Archives of Scientific Psychology, 6*(1), 63–69. https://doi.org/10.1037/arc0000043

Sabin, J. A., Marini, M., & Nosek, B. A. (2012). Implicit and explicit anti-fat bias among a large sample of medical doctors by BMI, race/ethnicity and gender. *PloS One, 7*(11), e48448. https://doi.org/10.1371/journal.pone.0048448

Setchell, J., Watson, B. M., Gard, M., & Jones, L. (2016). Physical therapists' ways of talking about overweight and obesity: Clinical implications. *Physical Therapy, 96*(6), 865–875. doi: https://doi.org/10.2522/ptj.20150286

Tomiyama, A. J., Carr, D., Granberg, E. M., Major, B., Robinson, E., Sutin, A. R., & Brewis, A. (2018). How and why weight stigma drives the obesity "epidemic" and harms health. *BMC Medicine, 16*(1), 1–6. https://doi.org/10.1186/s12916-018-1116-5

Tortelli, B. (2016, September 14). *The fear of discrimination in LGBT healthcare.* Institute for Public Health. https://publichealth.wustl.edu/fear-discrimination-lgbt-healthcare/

Tylka, T. L., Annunziato, R. A., Burgard, D., Daníelsdóttir, S., Shuman, E., Davis, C., & Calogero, R. M. (2014). The weight-inclusive versus weight-normative approach to health: Evaluating the evidence for prioritizing well-being over weight loss. *Journal of Obesity, 2014*, Article 983495. https://doi.org/10.1155/2014/983495

Wee, C. C., McCarthy, E. P., Davis, R. B., & Phillips, R. S. (2000). Screening for cervical and breast cancer: Is obesity an unrecognized barrier to preventive care? *Annals of Internal Medicine, 132*(9), 697–704. https://doi.org/10.7326/0003-4819-132-9-200005020-00003

Whitworth, H. B. Jr. (2017a). The challenge of noncompliance with medical recommendations, part 1. *MagMutual.* https://www.magmutual.com/learning/article/challenge-noncompliance-medical-recommendations-part-1/

Whitworth, H. B., Jr. (2017b). The challenge of noncompliance with medical recommendations, part 2. *MagMutual.* https://www.magmutual.com/learning/article/challenge-noncompliance-medical-recommendations-part-2/

Williams, J. C. (2017, August 24). Black Americans don't trust our healthcare system—here's why. *The Hill.* https://thehill.com/blogs/pundits-blog/healthcare/347780-black-americans-dont-have-trust-in-our-healthcare-system

Zolnierek, K. B. H., & DiMatteo, M. R. (2009). Physician communication and patient adherence to treatment: A meta-analysis. *Medical Care, 47*(8), 826–834. https://doi.org/10.1097/MLR.0b013e31819a5acc

Part II

Fattening pedagogy

Introduction
Heather A. Brown

In many ways, espousing Fat Studies within health professions education can feel a bit like denying climate change. After all, "obesity" is an epidemic. Here in the United States, both the Centers for Disease Control and the National Institutes of Health are invested in ending "obesity." The World Health Organization (n.d.) is likewise concerned, calling for the end of "globesity" on a webpage featuring a banner of a moderately heavy, fair-skinned, presumably Western man's headless torso with the buttons of his shirt gaping due to his bulk; this man—naturally—is eating that trendy avocado toast. The American Medical Association declared "obesity" a disease in 2013, and medical offices are now regularly paid (and often required by insurance companies) to address weight with clients (Hobbes, 2018).

Indeed, the medical profession is publicly and loudly concerned about the health of fat individuals.

> It is not a matter of benign padding. Compared to those with a normal or healthy weight, people who are obese face increased risk for dying of all causes and, more specifically, for suffering cardiovascular disease, type 2 diabetes, stroke, osteoarthritis, sleep apnea, certain cancers (20 percent of cancers in women and 16 percent in men are related to obesity), depression and anxiety, and many other chronic health complications. (Drexler, 2017, para. 6)

No citations are provided for this list of ailments, as if these statements are general common knowledge, although, in fact, they are often contested or at least challenged as being oversimplifications (O'Hara & Taylor, 2018). Still, those who will be entering the health professions are educated within this dominant "obesity" paradigm.

Current pedagogical focus

What are future health care professionals taught? What is the pedagogical focus of education about nutrition, diet, weight, and health? Unfortunately, the answer is "not much."

DOI: 10.4324/9781003057000-9

Hobbes (2018) reported on a 2015 survey of medical schools which found that their students received about 5 hours of education on nutrition annually over the course of a 4-year program. In general, medical schools are recommended to offer a minimum of 25 hours of education on the topic, but almost 40% offer less than half of that recommended amount (Adams et al., 2015). Such limited education can hardly begin to address any nutrition-effected illnesses (Adams et al., 2015; Butsch et al., 2020; Mastrocola et al., 2020).

Education on "obesity" is generally lumped in with nutrition education, although there have been some calls for specific "obesity"-focused education as well so that doctors and other health care professionals can be more effective in fighting fatness. Mastrocola et al. (2020), for example, argue that anti-"obesity" education should be required for both premed and medical students to that patients with "obesity" get the best possible treatment, while Butsch et al. (2020) found that medical students receive an "adequate" education on some issues related to "obesity" but that at least one-third of medical schools did not have any specific "obesity" education program and were unlikely to implement any in the future. The focus of that education was also of concern for Butsch et al. (2020) in that issues like communication with patients were not covered.

Several other studies also focused on the lack of knowledge about "obesity" but, as opposed to more general surveys about the state of "obesity" education, they instead focused on ways to improve the knowledge of both current and future health care professionals. Katz et al. (2005) argued for regular continuing education workshops to improve the confidence of family practitioners as well as their motivation to treat "obesity." Peters et al. (2013) found that medical students were actually over-confident in their knowledge of "obesity" but lacked the ability to integrate evidence-based theory into their communication practices with patients.

Other researchers have opted for a more "hands-on" approach to educate future health care professionals about "obesity." In one program, students were given extra credit for participating in "obesity educational interventions" including "a personal weight management experience that spanned at least 4 weeks, included calculations of body mass index (BMI), waist circumference, caloric needs, description of eating and physical activity and monitoring plan, and a final report and reflection" (Schmidt et al., 2013, p. 572). Schmidt et al. reported that, with little faculty time commitment, students could "see the effects on their own health while developing empathy for and understanding of the weight management struggles of their patients" (p. 572). Cotugna and Mallick (2010) also tested "a calorie restricted diet for 1 week (1,200 calories and 1,500 calories for women and men, respectively" to see if participating in a diet would promote empathy among dietetic and health promotion students (p. 321). They found that dieting did, indeed, effect a change in attitudes about fat people and argued that it "may be useful to incorporate this type of activity into the training of nutrition and other health professional students to increase sensitivity and reduce existing biases and negative attitudes toward overweight/obese clients" (Cotugna & Mallick, 2010, p. 321). Of course, these activities were promoted among learners without any consideration of the possibility that they could exacerbate any disordered eating already experienced by the students.

Finding ways to promote empathy and compassion for "people with obesity" and remove weight stigma has become an important component of "obesity" education for future health care professionals. Forhan and Salas (2013) argue, for example, that

> To address the inequities in obesity treatment it is imperative that weight bias be acknowledged and addressed. Without such actions weight bias will continue to negatively influence obesity treatment and unnecessarily impair the health and well-being of patients with obesity. (p. 207)

Indeed, there are many studies and even whole workshops and programmatic offerings that address trying to eradicate weight bias in current and future health care professionals. For example, Kushner et al. (2014) conducted a study in which the goal was to improve medical students' ability to communicate with an "overweight" standardized patient. A standardized patient is, in essence, a trained actor who provides an opportunity for future doctors to practice their skills in a simulated training environment (Johns Hopkins Medicine, n.d.). Students in Kushner et al.'s study read two articles on communication and stigma and were told to discuss the standardized patient's weight with them. Kushner et al. found some increases in empathy and lowering of bias in the short-term, but long-term results found the future health care professionals reverting to belief in stereotypes about "overweight" patients. What may be most interesting, however, is that among the six different scenarios the standardized patients were trained to use, each is grounded in the dominant "obesity" paradigm (see Kushner et al., 2014, p. 3 for the table). In none of them can the doctor and the patient have an interaction that is not grounded in the pursuit of weight loss.

In another, more recent, study, family medicine residents took part in a program in which they wore a "bariatric empathy suit" in order to develop empathy and compassion for "people living with obesity" (Luig et al., 2020). In fact, medical education programs designed to promulgate empathy and compassion through the use of what should be called "fat suits" has increased in recent years (Meadows et al., 2017). Meadows et al. argue, however, that such practices could not only backfire but also are highly unethical. Indeed, in popular culture, fat suits are often used as a form of mockery, sexism, and racism (Gullage, 2014; LeBesco, 2005; Mendoza, 2009). That a co-editor of *The Fat Pedagogy Reader*, Erin Cameron, who ought to know the damage that fat suits cause—even if you call them "bariatric empathy suits"—participated in the design and implementation of Luig et al.'s (2020) education program using them to promote empathy among future medical practitioners speaks to the difficulties inherent in challenging the dominant "obesity" paradigm in health care professions education.

Fat pedagogy

While many of the examples I have provided in this overview focus specifically on medical students or those areas that are most traditionally thought of in terms of "patient care," the same dominant discourse affects all caring professions, as demonstrated in the first section of this book. However, many individuals work-ing in those caring professions see—first hand in their own lives or in their own practices—how dangerous that dominant discourse can be to fat individuals and are taking steps to expand their learning and change the way they work—and to make suggestions for how the next generation of health care professionals can do better. They recognize that "weight-based oppression is a serious problem and that education is an important form of intervention" (Russell & Cameron, 2016, p. 252). Since the current pedagogy for future health care professionals is pri-marily grounded in dominant "obesity" discourse where weight loss is the focus, ignoring the evidence which finds that dieting does not work for over 90% of people (as discussed in our introduction) and since weight bias is problematic to fat individuals' health outcomes, what are the alternatives? How can we institute a pedagogy that is not just training future health care professionals to do more than find kinder and more compassionate ways to suggesting that fat people work harder at not being fat?

In the conclusion of their edited collection, *The Fat Pedagogy Reader,* Russell and Cameron (2016) have drafted a "manifesto" of what fat pedagogy is and how it must function. Fat pedagogy must:

- Shed light on weight bias and its pernicious effects;
- Engage in a scholar-practitioner method and/or dialogue in which academics and those in practice work with and inform each other's work;
- Be based on the lived experiences of individuals in fat bodies; and,
- Be generous and open, acknowledging that individuals expressing weight bias are not just "foolish and hateful," but exist—as we all do—in a fat-hating world that reinforces bias and discrimination in a systemic way (Russell & Cameron, 2016, p. 255)

Above all else, fat pedagogy must be used to make life better for fat people.

In many ways, fat pedagogy and the current pedagogy delineated by the domi-nant "obesity" paradigm are not entirely at odds—and if we take as the ultimate goal the concept that our work is to make the lives of fat people better, we share a common focus. Current pedagogy in health care professions acknowledges and is trying to address weight bias in its learners so they can be more compassionate and effective practitioners. Practice informs theory, and theory informs practice. Both pedagogies acknowledge that we live in a highly problematic world filled with systemic oppression and discrimination. And the work, even in the current pedagogy, is at least somewhat grounded in the lived experiences of fat individu-als, as the current paradigm works to understand and address how weight-based oppression and discrimination harms fat individuals. Where we disagree is what it means that our pedagogy helps make life better for fat individuals.

Ward and McPhail (2019) argue that we must "challenge existing fat hatred in both health care and the educational institutions that are so influential in shap-ing the care of those who interact with reproductive care professionals" (p. 265). While they were addressing their own profession, their statement applies to all health care professionals. The authors of the chapters in this section take Ward and McPhail's challenge to heart, while also demonstrating the important tenets of fat pedagogy as defined by Russell and Cameron (2016).

References

Adams, K. M., Butsch, W. S., & Kohlmeier, M. (2015). The state of nutrition education at US medical schools. *Journal of Biomedical Education*. Article ID 357627. https://doi. org/10.1155/2015/357627

Butsch, W. S., Kushner, R. F., Alford, S., & Smolarz, B. G. (2020). Low priority of obesity education leads to lack of medical students' preparedness to effectively treat patients with obesity: Results from the US medical school obesity education curriculum benchmark study. *BMC Medical Education, 20*(1), 23. https://doi.org/10.1186/s12909-020-1925-z

Cotugna, N., & Mallick, A. (2010). Following a calorie-restricted diet may help in reducing healthcare students' fat-phobia. *Journal of Community Health, 35*(3), 321–324. https://doi.org/10.1007/s10900-010-9226-9

Drexler, M. (2017). Obesity: Can we stop the epidemic? [Special report.] *Harvard Public Health: Magazine of the T. H. Chan School of Public Health.* https://www.hsph.harvard. edu/magazine/magazine_article/obesity/

Forhan, M., & Salas, X. R. (2013). Inequities in healthcare: A review of bias and discrimination in obesity treatment. *Canadian Journal of Diabetes, 37*(3), 205–209. https://doi. org/10.1016/j.jcjd.2013.03.362

Gullage, A. (2014). Fat Monica, fat suits, and *Friends*: Exploring narratives of fatness. *Feminist Media Studies, 14*(2), 178–189. https://doi.org/10.1080/14680777.2012.724026

Hobbes, M. (2018, September 19). *Everything you know about obesity is wrong*. Highline. https:// highline.huffingtonpost.com/articles/en/everything-you-know-about-obesity-is-wrong/

Johns Hopkins Medicine. (n.d.). Simulation Center. https://www.hopkinsmedicine.org/ simulation_center/training/standardized_patient_program/

Katz, S., Feigenbaum, A., Pasternak, S., & Vinker, S. (2005). An interactive course to enhance self-efficacy of family practitioners to treat obesity. *BMC Medical Education, 5*(4), 1–8. https://doi.org/10.1186/1472-6920-5-4

Kushner, R. F., Zeiss, D. M., Feinglass, J. M., & Yelen, M. (2014). An obesity educational intervention for medical students addressing weight bias and communication skills using standardized patients. *BMC Medical Education, 14*(53), 1–8. http://www. biomedcentral.com/1472-6920/14/53

LeBesco, K. (2005). Situating fat suits: Blackface, drag, and the politics of performance. *Women & Performance: A Journal of Feminist Theory, 15*(2), 231–242. https://doi. org/10.1080/07407700508571513

Luig, T., Wicklum, S., Heatherington, M., Vu, A., Cameron, E., Klein, D., Sharma, A. M., & Campbell-Scherer, D. L. (2020). Improving obesity management training in family medicine: Multi-methods evaluation of the 5AsT-MD pilot course. *BMC Medical Education, 20*(5). https://doi.org/10.1186/s12909-019-1908-0

Mastrocola, M. R., Roque, S. S., Benning, L. V., & Stanford, F. C. (2020). Obesity education in medical schools, residencies, and fellowships throughout the world: A systematic review. *International Journal of Obesity, 44*(2), 269–279. https://doi.org/10.1038/ s41366-019-0453-6

Meadows, A., Calogero, R., O'Reilly, C., Rodriguez, A. C. I., Heldreth, C. M., & Tomiyama, A. J. (2017). Why fat suits do not advance the scientific study of weight stigma. *Obesity, 25*(2), 275. https://doi.org/10.1002/oby.21742

Mendoza, K. R. (2009). Seeing through the layers: Fat suits and thin bodies in "The Nutty Professor" and "Shallow Hal." In E. Rothblum & S. Solovay (Eds.), *The fat studies reader* (pp. 280–288). New York University Press.

O'Hara, L., & Taylor, J. (2018). What's wrong with the "war on obesity?" A narrative review of the weight-centered health paradigm and development of the 3C framework to build critical competency for a paradigm shift. *Sage Open*, 8(2). https://doi.org/10.1177/2158244018772888

Peters, S., Bird, L., Ashraf, H., Ahmed, S., McNamee, P., Ng, C., & Hart, J. (2013). Medical undergraduates' use of behaviour change talk: The example of facilitating weight management. *BMC Medical Education*, 13(7), 1–12. http://www.biomedcentral.com/1472-6920/13/7

Russell, C., & Cameron, E. (2016). Conclusion: A fat pedagogy manifesto. In E. Cameron & C. Russell (Eds.), *The fat pedagogy reader: Challenging weight-based oppression through critical education* (pp. 251–256). Peter Lang.

Schmidt, S., Rice, A., & Kolasa, K. (2013). Teaching by example—Educating medical students through a weight management experience. *Family Medicine*, 45(8), 572–575.

Ward, P., & McPhail, D. (2019). A shared vision for reducing fat shame and blame in reproductive care. *Women's Reproductive Health*, 6(4), 265–270. https://doi.org/10.1080/23293691.2019.1653582

World Health Organization. (n.d.). *Controlling the global obesity epidemic*. https://www.who.int/activities/controlling-the-global-obesity-epidemic

8 Raising awareness of weight-based oppression in health care

Reflections on lived experience education as emotional labor

Sara Martel, Alex Andrews, Laura Griffin, Amanda Hollahan, Sonia Meerai, May Friedman, Christine Heidebrecht, Chelsea D'Silva, Dianne Fierheller, and Ian Zenlea

The pilot project discussed in this chapter is a collaboration between lived experience educators (Alex, Laura, Amanda, Sonia), researchers (Chelsea, May, Christine, Sara), practicing clinicians (Dianne, Ian), and a medical learner (Helia). Together, we are creating a series of podcasts that share insights into lived experiences with weight-based oppression in health care settings. The podcasts will be shared with a sample of hospital-based physicians and nurses to listen to and reflect on. The health care providers will then come together in a 1-hour workshop to further engage with the content in a safe and open forum for dialogue. Participants will complete a questionnaire after they listen to each podcast and an interview 6-months after workshop completion to discuss how or if the podcasts and workshop informed their attitudes, beliefs, or practices in any way. The learning generated through this pilot is intended to inform future iterations of the content and design, which we hope to build into curriculum.

Although the realities of weight-based bias, stigmatization, and discrimination in health care settings are well-documented (Ellison et al., 2016; Greenhalgh, 2012; Herndon, 2014; McNaughton & Smith, 2016; Pausé, 2014; Puhl & Heuer, 2010; Puhl & Suh, 2015; Wilson, 2009), research on how to best address these issues remains slight (Alberga et al., 2016). It is also rare to see the language of "oppression" in existing literature, though that is the framework we propose as most appropriate (Prohaska & Gailey, 2019). We hope our work serves to mitigate the lack of theoretical frameworks for weight-based oppression within existing health profession education. Educators face the pedagogical challenge of teaching scientifically trained professionals to deconstruct the discursive "war on obesity" that has been waged through the medicalization of fat bodies (Greenhalgh, 2012; Thille et al., 2017). For systemic change to emerge, health professionals need to be able to locate their personal biases within structural conditions—a point

DOI: 10.4324/9781003057000-10

overlooked in the current literature that focuses on competency building but not consciousness raising (Alberga et al., 2016). The field of Fat Studies has yielded copious amounts of scholarship to support systemic transformation of these realities (for example see Russell, 2020; Wann, 2009), yet is strikingly silent in health profession education.

Collectively, we recognize that education can reproduce existing power relations by reinforcing dominant cultural and social roles (Freire, 2005). Democratic and emancipatory education must involve those who experience oppression in the process of understanding and transforming the conditions that shape their lives. We argue a vital aspect of fattening pedagogy is ensuring fat communities, are not further objectified or othered by curriculum designed externally to their own lived experience. This tenet bears the significance of lived experience in education as a fundamental aspect of our study design.

The concept of teaching and learning through lived experience runs throughout social justice education (Charlton, 2000; Dewey, 1916; Freire, 2005). Health care is also beginning to promote lived experience as a valuable form of knowledge and expertise (Dorozenko et al., 2016; Gilbert & Stickley, 2012; Happell et al., 2015; Happell et al., 2014; Meehan & Glover, 2007; Meeks & Jain, 2018). The inclusion of individuals who have lived experience in co-design and advisory roles has shown to promote better care, improve health outcomes, and support the development of interpersonal skills, compassion and empathy, while challenging stigma, bias and discrimination (Dorozenko et al., 2016; Happell et al., 2015; Happell et al., 2014; Meehan & Glover, 2007).

But what does it mean to self-author oneself as a lived experience educator within the very health care system that imposes one's oppression? What does it mean to tell one's story not of illness but of the suffering under discrimination of fat bodies? How do we both deconstruct the power relations that produce the "obese patient" (Friedman, 2012; Medvedyuk et al., 2018; Moffat, 2010), while inviting educators to speak from their authority as those who live in fat bodies? These are some of the questions this chapter explores through critical and personal reflections on the role of lived experience education in our own project. Ultimately, we offer insight into lived experience education as a form of emotional labor (Hochschild, 1979, 1983). We hope this writing serves to inform future work that gives voice to lived experience as a vital aspect of fattening pedagogy, while also illuminating its contours, challenges, and advantages in order to understand the politics of this pedagogical work.

Study overview: This project's story

At the time of writing this chapter, the lived experience educators have all completed recording sessions facilitated by May. The general themes covered in the sessions emerged through previous meetings with the educators and some research team members, providing general touch-points to guide the discussions. This raw content will be collaboratively edited into multiple episodes over the next few months. Recruitment for the study is anticipated to take place in the Fall of 2021.

While our study is still ongoing, we offer insights of our work-to-date from a process of self-reflexivity—the active and reflective processes of paying attention to our epistemological values and our positions within the context of this work (Alvesson & Sköldberg, 2009; Haraway, 1991; Harding, 2004; Pausé, 2020). We all contribute from our positions within interdisciplinary, interprofessional, and diverse social identities, collaborating from inside our experiences of weight-based oppression or our experiences of thin privilege. As a collaborative research-creation team, our shared understanding about health care's anti-fat problematic is born in different ways. The lived experience educators among us are taking on an incredible amount of vulnerability to improve a system within which we have experienced oppression. Those of us who are learners are grappling with how to become weight inclusive clinicians while being trained within a system that exclusively promotes a weight normative model of care. Those of us who are practicing providers and researchers are exploring and challenging our own complicity in anti-fat oppression by the nature of our knowledges and practices. As members of many different communities, we are all attempting to contribute to a social justice movement toward fat acceptance, equity, and equality that we believe must include significant changes in health care to be achieved and sustained.

The clinicians on the team, Ian and Dianne, became aware of the impacts of weight bias, stigma, and discrimination while working alongside children and their families in a pediatric weight management program. Within this "professional knowledge landscape" (Clandinin & Connelly, 1996), stories and experiences of fatness were lived, told and retold everyday by children, youth, caregivers, siblings, and clinicians. Many individuals shared their unique experiences of weight bias, stigma, and discrimination throughout the many spaces of their lives, including health care (Zenlea et al., 2017). Stories were told of judgement, shame, blame, hurt, and interrogation, but also of beauty, strength, resilience, acceptance, and love. While health care aims to "help" individuals, the systemic discrimination directed toward fat bodies is very present and has significant impacts. The grand narrative that fatness is "unhealthy" and requires "intervention" is woven throughout the clinic and the institutional policies that guide practices.

As Ian and Dianne sat alongside individuals and families listening to these stories, they began to reflect on their own practices and ways of knowing as clinicians and researchers. Learning from the experiential knowledge of fat children and their families, we wondered how we could start to make shifts within our clinical practices that would promote health and health equity for all bodies. We began to envision collaborations with other researchers as well as ways to highlight the voices of those experiencing bias and stigma firsthand.

From here an interdisciplinary team grew to include researchers from critical Fat Studies (May), media and cultural studies (Sara), anthropology and epidemiology (Christine), and health systems research (Chelsea). Helia also joined as a research assistant and medical student grappling with the explicit and implicit anti-fat values that she has recognized as being built into pedagogical environments and curriculum. We began with the idea that storytelling could be a powerful way to raise awareness of weight-based oppression in health care set-tings among care-providers. Narrative knowledge provides an alternative way of knowing to the positivist epistemologies that characterize the field of science and medicine (Charon, 2001, 2006; Frank, 1995). Rather than reducing people to their biomedical facts, stories can open up storytellers and listeners alike to a rich world of nuance, paradox, struggle, joy, and all the other complexities of living in our bodies as "patients." Medical education frequently calls on narrative as a means for communicating lived experience in order to promote self-reflection and empathy (Cox, 2001; Easton, 2016; Haigh & Hardy, 2011). There is also evidence of therapeutic benefits for patients who share their stories (Jackson et al., 2003; Player et al., 2019). Translating lived experience into narrative structure is a pow-erful form of self-authorship, inviting story-tellers into sense-making and teaching as more than objects of study (Benmayor, 2008; Rodriguez, 2010).

What is foundational to the project's story and to the ideas we offer in this chapter, however, is that the stories needing to be told are not about illness expe-riences but about experiences of oppression within health care. Many of the orig-inal researchers live in thin bodies and are aware these stories of oppression are not theirs to tell. Although all of us as co-authors can claim the "authenticity" of our own experiences, our collective goal is to center the voices of those among us who have been systemically marginalized (i.e., patients who live in fat bodies), not those who have been systemically privileged (i.e., clinicians and researchers work-ing within dominant narratives of thinness and health; Applebaum, 2008). The original team members reached out across various scholarly networks to recruit individuals who would be interested in collaborating on this project as lived expe-rience educators. Alex, Laura, Amanda, and Sonia all joined the team and have led the content development and production of the podcasts. Our collaboration has been conceived within participatory principles (Israel et al., 2010; Wallerstein & Duran, 2006), which aim to recognize all team members as equal and equitable partners in knowledge production. Many of the theoretical insights shared in this chapter have derived from hours of discussion about not only their personal experiences but their critical perspectives as emerging scholars.

The emotional labor of teaching and learning from lived experience

Our project is based on the idea that lived experience is pedagogical: it has something to say if we give it language and has something to teach if we give it reflection. We trace the concept of lived experience through phenomenology, which is a branch of philosophy interested in understanding how experiences are brought to consciousness—in other words how we live phenomena in the world as embodied and affective agents (Ahmed, 2006; Kruks, 2014; van Manen, 2015). Lived experience teaches others about phenomena from within. It provides a sense of not only what a thing *is* but what it *feels like*. We specify the provision of *a* sense and not *the* sense in recognition that there is no essential experience. There is no singular way to communicate one's lived experience or singular way for a learner to interpret the communication. In all of these ways, teaching and learning with lived experience is an active, subjective, embodied, and fluid process of sense-making.

We heed the feminist critique that a politics based on "authentic" experience overlooks the role of ideology in producing the way we know and move through the world (Scott, 1991). Developing theoretically sound pedagogy requires we think through the role of language, material conditions, and cultural frameworks in shaping our lived experiences. Stories can serve to reinforce rather than dismantle existing power relations, particularly the privileging of some stories over others. Within this project we have wrestled constantly with questions of representation and for whom our experience may and may not speak; to neglect such questions is to neglect the intersectionality of fatness with racialized, gendered, ableist, and colonial politics of identity formation (Friedman et al., 2020). Speaking from her own self-identified position as a "person with lived experience," Voronka questions the risks for patients who must take on "a form of strategic essentialism" (Voronka, 2016, p. 190) in order to be recognized by health care as someone who can speak to certain experiences. We must ensure individuals are granted fluid and self-determined identities even as they are asked to embody a specific subjectivity from which they are expected to teach. As lived experience is constructed by health care as a form of expert knowledge, there is potential for its objectification; it becomes reified as capital that lived experience educators hold and health care organizations can leverage. This objectification risks distancing lived experience educators from their own experiences as something to possess and impart, rather than something felt or intersubjectively held between learners and teachers.

We offer the idea that conceptualizing lived experience education as emotional labor can mitigate the risk of objectification. Framing this form of teaching as labor helps challenge the notion that it depends on the fixed identity of the educator, rather than on a dynamic process of becoming through the work of self-authoring. Arlie Hochschild's foundational work defines emotional labor as the work of expressing and managing one's own emotions in order to produce an emotional state in others (Hochschild, 1979, 1983). In the context of the lived experience educators among us, we acknowledge there is work to speaking our truth while recognizing it will challenge those who are actors in the system of our oppression. There is work in knowing our experience of oppression is also our assertion of authority. There is work to holding ourselves in a space that balances vulnerability and expertise. There is work in holding the fluidity and self-determination of our own identities with the need to embody the experience of fatness.

Our project's pedagogical objective is not only to foster compassion among health care professionals and learners but engender a questioning of their beliefs and assumptions about fatness, fat bodies, and weight-based oppression. We draw on a "pedagogy of discomfort" (Boler, 1999) as a teaching practice "grounded in the assumption that discomforting feelings are important in challenging dominant beliefs, social habits and normative practices that sustain social inequities as they create openings for individual and social transformation" (Zembylas, 2015, p. 163). While a pedagogy of discomfort focuses on the emotional and affective impact of social justice curriculum on learners, it is equally important to consider the emotional labor lived experience educators take on to generate that discomfort. This requires us to engage with the idea that a significant aspect of lived experience education is the labor of offering one's own stories of suffering (and resilience and empowerment and many other facets of experience) as teaching tools. We explore the dimensions of this labor in the section below through personal reflections offered by some of the authors.

What we've learned so far

Amanda (Lived Experience Educator)

From the onset of this project, I wanted to be mindful that my experience with weight-based discrimination within health care would not be the same as every fat person's experience, nor the same as my co-lived experienced educators' experience. We are all coming from unique positionalities with distinct, varied, and complicated relationships with fatness, and health care for that matter. What unites our team of lived experience educators is an understanding that the health care system, predominantly speaking, has failed fat folks. Whether this began during childhood, at the onset of a newly diagnosed health condition, or as an adult, all of us have experienced harm at the hands of those who were meant to explicitly help us.

With all of this in mind, being a part of this project began from a place of pain. Sitting in a doctor's office as a child, was the first time and place that I realized my body was wrong. Before I was even in control of all of the food I was eating, I was explicitly told that I was too big and that I needed to "watch" my weight. Please note, this is not me suggesting that the blame should have been shifted towards my parents, specifically my mother, but rather, an outcry for some compassion for a child who would now feel the need to shrink herself, when her body had not yet even finished growing. From that moment on, the doctor's office became a place I feared going, as it symbolized all the ways in which my body was perceived to be a failure.

The pain I brought into this project helped to motivate me, but it also made me cautious. The doctors and health care providers who had harmed me so viciously in the past, had not set out to cause harm. Quite the opposite, I can imagine. They were trying to do good, trying to help me, trying to make me "healthy." So, what was to say that the set of health care providers working on this study were any different?

While I was cautious entering this study, the team I worked with directly, as well as my fellow lived experience educators, made me feel like my pain and cautiousness were not only valid, but righteous. They listened and took notes and validated my feelings when I shared my problems with the health care system and the ways in which fat folks are marginalized by the equating of weight with health. They held space, listened to feedback and were, most importantly, willing to learn about what they could be doing better. Slowly my fear started to fade, and I began to get excited about the possibility of something wonderful and meaningful emerging from this project and our podcasts.

Again, this is not to say that we did not have concerns about how to formulate our podcasts, or fears surrounding the ways in which our experiences would be perceived by the health care professionals who listened to them. We had many discussions surrounding the best way to formulate the podcasts, or most efficient way of phrasing our experiences, out of fear that our knowledge could be dismissed as anecdotal. While many of us work and learn within academic spaces, we wanted to be mindful that our knowledge as lived experience educators should not have to be substantiated, in order to matter. Our lived experiences were, in fact, the basis for our knowledge. With this in mind, we decided that our experiences, fears, anger, and pain were all valid and all worth including within the podcasts.

When we finally recorded our first set of audios, I came to the recording with this framework in mind. I did not prepare or write anything in advance, and instead set out to speak from a place of honesty. While the final episodes have not been edited or released at the point of writing this, the majority of my segments have been recorded, and while I am glad that my experiences and voice were included in this project, I am also left feeling cautious once again.

Though I am proud of the work I have put into this project and I stand behind everything I and my fellow lived experience educators have said, I am nervous. Nervous that our experiences will not be taken seriously. Anxious that our histories of mistreatment within health care will be dismissed as outlier cases. Fearful that our words could somehow be turned against us, in some sort of twisted "gotcha" moment. And most of all, I am scared that we are not doing or saying enough.

But I am also hopeful. Hopeful that this project and the podcasts we produce will make a difference. Hopeful that the health care professionals who listen to them, or the people that read this article, understand that weight and fatness are not intrinsically linked to poor health or poor health outcomes. Hopeful, that at the very least, health care professionals will start asking basic questions that prioritize their patients physical and emotional wellbeing. Hopeful that these podcasts have an impact and health care professionals become more willing to sit in their own discomfort for the betterment of those they treat.

Laura (Lived Experience Educator)

I would like to start off by saying that sharing my experience as a fat person in a health care setting is both liberating and emotionally draining. The continuous positionality of having to be a fat person that has to advocate for themselves is emotional labor. The most difficult part about it is that we are advocating that we be treated with respect, kindness, support and ultimately, love. To be put in a position that has to present ourselves as someone who should be acknowledged or that our existence should be acknowledged with support and love is ultimately where the tension between fat person and health care worker begins. This tension is both personal and institutional because it is grounded in the idea that fat people do not deserve respect from health care professions. Thus, using our stories in a podcast platform, will hopefully put a humanistic perspective behind the words of a medical textbook that speaks on obesity—every time you see that word, interact with it, there is a human being that is impacted by it. The opportunity to speak directly into the ears of health care professionals will hopefully be a step towards changing how they interact with fat patients but also interrogate the emotional labor that fat people take on in order to be treated respectfully.

Internalized fatphobia will always be present. As mentioned in the podcast, it's a hard dichotomy between 'yes body positivity' and 'no, I actually hate my body.' There is so much emotional labor and work that fat people have to individually do in regard to loving their own self yet absolutely no work is being done from society, or even health care settings to also establish self-love. Even within a body positive movement, there will be internalized fatphobia because you may want to love yourself, but the world does not, and it will continue to show you why you should not.

We need to see the intersection of fat bodies with biomedical training; this means, fat doctors and the interaction of fat literature in medical school settings. There is already fat literature, research and projects being done in regard to obesity and its impact. This type of work needs to be intersected in medical spaces. This could be done by putting pressure to form allyship, meaning a collaborative movement, a movement of all body sizes in solidarity with fat bodies. But honestly, we need to start simply respecting fat bodies, and we are not there yet. Which will make this particular intersectionality of biomedical training and fatness difficult. If we don't even love Fat bodies yet, how do we really show the respect needed in medical spaces.

Alex (Lived Experience Educator)

I joined this study because I saw how much both my community and I were being impacted by medicalized fat phobia. Sharing and reflecting on my interactions with physicians and the health care system has been a very vulnerable experience for me due to multiple negative interactions. I am hoping that through sharing my experiences I can help to challenge the way fat people are stigmatized in medical settings. It is therefore very important that doctors are familiar with the different forms of discrimination that are occurring in their profession. This way they have the option of learning to do better by their fat patients.

Health care providers need to be aware of using words like body mass index (BMI) and obesity when the context is not correct. They also need to be aware of their power dynamic and the impact that their words have in response to weight. For example, it is very important that a doctor does not conflate patient health issues with obesity. Multiple accounts have shown that this leads to alienation of the patient or, worse, death, because something was written off as being caused only by obesity. These words have meaning and I wish that there was a way to make doctors do anti fat discrimination training. Since that is not a current reality as an option, this podcast is an option to speak directly to doctors.

In our meetings, we talked about gender affirming surgery and the problematic way it has been used by medical practitioners as a roadblock. In my case, it is important that doctors learn how harmful it is to use BMI as a roadblock to gender affirming surgery. I have been told over and over to lose weight in order to get the surgeries that I need to reflect who I am. In order to get a gender affirming surgery, either top surgery or bottom surgery, you have to reach a certain number on the BMI scale. Since it has been proven that BMI is an outdated and racist measure, it does not make sense that medical professionals still use this as a bureaucratic barrier. I would love to be able to share this, in hope that even just one health care provider changes their mind.

Sonia (Lived Experience Educator)
I am a fat, racialized woman. My experiences within the Ontario health care system have been complicated, alarming, and etched in survival—rather, surviving how to navigate its complexities of health care provider biases and assumptions which I have observed, experienced, and researched about when working with BIPOC (Black, Indigenous, and People of Color) communities who are bigger than the constructed "norm." The project allowed for a safe space to discuss and disrupt common assumptions and violent practices which have been experienced. Specifically, I traced my health care experience from childhood to present day, connecting it to different health care provider spaces such as the family health team, hospital, speciality clinics, and emergent care. The main learnings from my reflective process post-recording the podcast was that I focused on the utility of BMI and how it is used as a form of being dismissed and ignored in health care-based conversations with health care providers—from my standpoint. I ended my podcast recording with a kind of critical hope—a hope that more humanness be embedded in health care provider practices when they too, must navigate their protocols and procedures in providing care and thinking through their impact beyond the numbers.

Helia (Medical Student)
As a medical student on this project, with every encounter and story, and by immersing myself in disciplines like critical Fat Studies, I learned more about the qualities that make a good physician. I was the only medical representative in the lived experience discussion meetings, and this was followed with a lot of heartbreak and learning. The lived experience educators mentioned stories where many 'overweight' individuals no longer felt safe seeking care, and the doctor's office had become a space of fear rather than a space they can go to in the face of health vulnerability. This came as a shock, as this subject is far from prioritized in medical education, yet its impacts seem to be overwhelming. Being involved in this project has taught me that the medicalization of those who live in larger bodies and the insidiously negative discourse on obesity has created an atmosphere of weight-bias that is detrimental to patient care.

Listening to each experience of exclusion and fat-shaming bore with it an intense heartbreak and an overpowering responsibility for the wrong doings. I internalized every word and allowed my strong emotion to permanently shape my identity as a future physician. The lived experience educators have taught me how to best talk about sensitive issues, how to follow the lead of my patient and how to create a partnership where my patient feels safe to come to me with anything. They have gifted me the knowledge of the patient perspective, in an environment that allowed them to feel safe and heard. From my experience with this project, and now being in my clinical year of medicine, the significance of the social determinants is immensely pronounced and failure to acknowledge this is detrimental. No matter the path I take in my medical journey, I will create a weight inclusive practice and strive to be an individual that helps lift the burden of health vulnerability through a multisystemic approach with special attention to the impacts of the social determinants of health. I will commit to a life of continuous learning from those with lived experience, although many times it can feel emotionally heavy, so I can be the best physician for my patients.

Concluding remarks

Our project explores the potential for lived experience education and storytelling to help raise awareness amongst health professionals about weight-based oppression. We argue that lived experience education ought to play a vital role in the deconstruction of fatness in health care as it currently stands and the reconstruction of equitable and weight-inclusive knowledges and practices in its place. For this reason, we need to understand the pedagogical, political, and theoretical dimensions of educating through one's experience of fatness in health care, while being sure not to empty it out of its personal and emotional power as a form of self-authorship. Striking such a balance is key to building support for lived experience educators in meaningful ways and ensuring health profession education does not reproduce the very power relations we are striving to disrupt by fattening pedagogy.

References

Ahmed, S. (2006). *Queer phenomenology: Orientations, objects, others*. Duke University Press.

Alberga, A. S., Pickering, B. J., Alix Hayden, K., Ball, G. D., Edwards, A., Jelinski, S., Nutter, S., Oddie, S., Sharma, A. M., & Russell-Mayhew, S. (2016). Weight bias reduction in health professionals: A systematic review. *Clinical Obesity*, 6(3), 175–188. https://doi.org/10.1111/cob.12147

Alvesson, M., & Sköldberg, K. (2009). *Reflexive methodology: New vistas for qualitative research* (2nd ed.). Sage.

Applebaum, B. (2008). "Doesn't my experience count?" White students, the authority of experience and social justice pedagogy. *Race Ethnicity and Education*, 11(4), 405–414. https://doi.org/10.1080/13613320802478945

Benmayor, R. (2008). Digital storytelling as a signature pedagogy for the new humanities. *Arts and Humanities in Higher Education*, 7(2), 188–204. https://doi.org/10.1177/1474022208088648

Boler, M. (1999). *Feeling power: Emotions and education*. Routledge.

Charlton, J. I. (2000). *Nothing about us without us: Disability oppression and empowerment*. University of California Press.

Charon, R. (2001). The patient-physician relationship. Narrative medicine: A model for empathy, reflection, profession, and trust. *JAMA*, 286(15), 1897–1902. https://doi.org/10.1001/jama.286.15.1897

Charon, R. (2006). *Narrative medicine: Honoring the stories of illness*. Oxford University Press.

Clandinin, D., & Connelly, F. (1996). Teachers' professional knowledge landscapes: Teacher stories—Stories of teachers—School stories—Stories of school. *Educational Researcher*, 25(3), 24–30 https://doi.or/10/3102/0013189X025003024

Cox, K. (2001). Stories as case knowledge: Case knowledge as stories. *Medical Education*, 35(9), 862–866. https://doi.org/10.1046/j.1365-2923.2001.01016.x

Dewey, J. (1916). *Democracy and education*. The Free Press.

Dorozenko, K. P., Ridley, S., Martin, R., & Mahboub, L. (2016). A journey of embedding mental health lived experience in social work education. *Social Work Education*, 35(8), 905–917. https://doi.org/10.1080/02615479.2016.1214255

Easton, G. (2016). How medical teachers use narratives in lectures: A qualitative study. *BMC Medical Education*, 16, 3. https://doi.org/10.1186/s12909-015-0498-8

Ellison, J., McPhail, D., & Mitchinson, W. (2016). Introduction: Obesity in Canada. In J. Ellison, D. McPhail, & W. Mitchinson (Eds.), *Obesity in Canada: Critical perspectives* (pp. 3–28). University of Toronto Press.

Frank, A. W. (1995). *The Wounded storyteller: Body, illness, and ethics*. The University of Chicago Press.

Freire, P. (2005). *Pedagogy of the oppressed: 30th anniversary edition*. The Continuum International Publishing Group, Inc.

Friedman, M. (2012). Fat is a social work issue: Fat bodies, moral regulation, and the history of social work. *Intersectionalities: A Global Journal of Social Work Analysis, Research, Policy and Practice*, 1, 53–69. https://journals.library.mun.ca/ojs/index.php/IJ/article/view/350

Friedman, M., Rice, C., & Rinaldi, J.. (Eds.). (2020). *Thickening fat: Fat bodies, intersectionality, and social justice*. Routledge.

Gilbert, P., & Stickley, T. (2012). "Wounded healers": The role of lived-experience in mental health education and practice. *The Journal of Mental Health Training, Education and Practice*, 7(1), 33–41. https://doi.org/10/1108/17556221211230570

Greenhalgh, S. (2012). Weighty subjects: The biopolitics of the U.S. war on fat. *American Ethnologist*, 39(3), 471–487. https://doi.org/10.1111/j.1548-1425.2012.01375.x

Haigh, C., & Hardy, P. (2011). Tell me a story—A conceptual exploration of storytelling in healthcare education. *Nurse Education Today*, 31(4), 408–411. https://doi.org/10.1016/j.nedt.2010.08.001

Happell, B., Bennetts, W., Harris, S., Platania-Phung, C., Tohotoa, J., Byrne, L., & Wynaden, D. (2015). Lived experience in teaching mental health nursing: Issues of fear and power. *International Journal of Mental Health Nursing*, 24(1), 19–27. https://doi.org/10.1111/inm.12091

Happell, B., Byrne, L., McAllister, M., Lampshire, D., Roper, C., Gaskin, C. J., Martin, G., Wynaden, D., McKenna, B., Lakeman, R., Platania-Phung, C., & Hamer, H. (2014). Consumer involvement in the tertiary-level education of mental health professionals: A systematic review. *International Journal of Mental Health Nursing*, 23(1), 3–16. https://doi.org/10.1111/inm.12021

Haraway, D. (1991). *Simians, cyborgs, and women: The reinvention of nature*. Routledge.

Harding, S. (2004). Introduction: Standpoint theory as a site of political, philosophical and scientific debate. In S. Harding (Ed.), *The feminist standpoint theory reader: Intellectual and political controversies* (pp. 1–16.). Routledge.

Herndon, A. (2014). *Fat blame: How the war on obesity victimizes women and children.* University Press of Kansas.

Hochschild, A. R. (1979). Emotion work, feeling rules, and social structure. *American Journal of Sociology, 85*(3), 551–575. https://doi.org/10.1086/227049

Hochschild, A. R. (1983). *The managed heart: Commercialization of human feeling.* University of California Press.

Israel, B. A., Coombe, C. M., Cheezum, R. R., Schulz, A. J., McGranaghan, R. J., Lichtenstein, R., Reyes, A. G., Clement, J., & Burris, A. (2010). Community-based participatory research: A capacity-building approach for policy advocacy aimed at eliminating health disparities. *American Journal of Public Health, 100*(11), 2094–2102. https://doi.org/10.2105/AJPH.2009.170506

Jackson, A., Blaxter, L., & Lewando-Hundt, G. (2003). Participating in medical education: Views of patients and carers living in deprived communities. *Medical Education, 37*(6), 532–538. https://doi.org/10.1046/j.1365-2923.2003.01535.x

Kruks, S. (2014). Women's "lived experience": Feminism and phenomenology from Simone de Beauvoir to the present. In M. Evans, C. Hemmings, M. Henry, H. Johnstone, S. Madhok, A. Plomien, & S. Wearing (Eds.), *The SAGE handbook of feminist theory.* SAGE.

McNaughton, D., & Smith, C. (2016). Diabesity, or the "twin epidemics": Reflections on the iatrogenic consequences of stigmatizing lifestyle to reduce the incidence of diabetes mellitus in Canada. In J. Ellison, D. McPhail, & W. Mitchinson (Eds.), *Obesity in Canada: Critical perspectives* (pp. 122–147). University of Toronto Press.

Medvedyuk, S., Ali, A., & Raphael, D. (2018). Ideology, obesity and the social determinants of health: A critical analysis of the obesity and health relationship. *Critical Public Health, 28*(5), 573–585. https://doi.org/10.1080/09581596.2017.1356910

Meehan, T., & Glover, H. (2007). Telling our story: Consumer perceptions of their role in mental health education. *Psychiatric Rehabilitation Journal, 31*(2), 152–154. https://doi.org/10.2975/31.2.2007.152.154

Meeks, L. M., & Jain, N. R. (2018). *Accessibility, inclusion and action in medical education: Lived experiences of learners and physicians with disabilities.* Association of American Medical Colleges. https://sds.ucsf.edu/sites/g/files/tkssra2986/f/aamc-ucsf-disability-special-report-accessible.pdf

Moffat, T. (2010). The "childhood obesity epidemic": Health crisis or social construction? *Medical Anthropology Quarterly, 24*(1), 1–21. https://doi.org/10.1111/j.1548-1387.2010.01082.x

Pausé, C. (2014). Die another day: The obstacles facing fat people in accessing quality healthcare. *Narrative Inquiry in Bioethics, 4*(2), 135–141. https://doi.org/10.1353/nib.2014.0039

Pausé, C. (2020). Ray of light: Standpoint theory. Fat Studies, and a new fat ethics. *Fat Studies, 9*(2), 175–187. https://doi.org/10.1080/21604851.2019.1630203

Player, E., Gure-Klinke, H., North, S., Hanson, S., Lane, D., Culyer, G., & Rodrigues, V. (2019). Humanising medicine: Teaching on tri-morbidity using expert patient narratives in medical education. *Education for Primary Care, 30*(6), 368–374. https://doi.org/10.1080/14739879.2019.1670097

Prohaska, A., & Gailey, J. A. (2019). Theorizing fat oppression: Intersectional approaches and methodological innovations. *Fat Studies, 8*(1), 1–9. https://doi.org/10.1080/21604851.2019.1534469

Puhl, R., & Heuer, C. A. (2010). Obesity stigma: Important considerations for public health. *American Journal of Public Health, 100*(6), 1019–1028. https://doi.org/10.2105/AJPH.2009.159491

Puhl, R., & Suh, Y. (2015). Health consequences of weight stigma: Implications for obesity prevention and treatment. *Current Obesity Reports*, 4(2), 182–190. https://doi.org/10.1007/s13679-015-0153-z

Rodriguez, D. (2010). Storytelling in the field: Race, method, and the empowerment of Latina college students. *Cultural Studies* ↔ *Critical Methodologies*, 10(6), 491–507. https://doi.org/10.1177/1532708610365481

Russell, C. (2020). Fat pedagogy and the disruption of weight-based oppression: Toward the flourishing of all bodies. In S. Steinberg & B. Down (Eds.), *The SAGE handbook of critical pedagogies* (pp. 1516–1531). Sage.

Scott, J. W. (1991). The evidence of experience. *Critical Inquiry*, 17(4), 773–797. http://www.jstor.org/stable/1343743

Thille, P., Friedman, M., & Setchell, J. (2017). Weight-related stigma and health policy. *CMAJ*, 189(6), e223–e224. https://doi.org/10.1503/cmaj.160975

van Manen, M. (2015). *Researching lived experience: Human science for an action sensitive pedagogy*. Routledge.

Voronka, J. (2016). The politics of "people with lived experience" experiential authority and the risks of strategic essentialism. *Philosophy, Psychiatry, & Psychology*, 23(3–4), 189–201. https://doi.org/10.1353/ppp.2016.0017

Wallerstein, N. B., & Duran, B. (2006). Using community-based participatory research to address health disparities. *Health Promotion Practice*, 7(3), 312–323. https://doi.org/10.1177/1524839906289376

Wann, M. (2009). Foreword: Fat studies: An invitation to revolution. In E. Rothblum & S. Solovay (Eds.), *The fat studies reader* (pp. ix–xxv). New York University Press.

Wilson, B. (2009). Widening the dialogue to narrow the gap in health disparities: Approaches to fat Black lesbian and bisexual women's health promotion. In E. Rothblum & S. Solovay (Eds.), *The fat studies reader* (pp. 54–64). New York University Press.

Zembylas, M. (2015). "Pedagogy of discomfort" and its ethical implications: The tensions of ethical violence in social justice education. *Ethics and Education*, 10(2), 163–174. https://doi.org/10.1080/17449642.2015.1039274

Zenlea, I. S., Thompson, B., Fierheller, D., Green, J., Ulloa, C., Wills, A., & Mansfield, E. (2017). Walking in the shoes of caregivers of children with obesity: Supporting caregivers in paediatric weight management. *Clinical Obesity*, 7(5), 300–306. https://doi.org/10.1111/cob.12202

9 The weight of imaginative resistance and pedagogy for narrative transformation

Elizabeth Lanphier and Hannah Cory

This chapter unpacks a thick description of one author's (Hannah Cory) personal narrative of her motivations to enter the field of nutrition and pivotal experiences during training. The first-person descriptions, which run throughout as offset text, are in conversation with the theoretical framing of imaginative resistance from philosophical literature, and the techniques of narrative medicine, engaged by the other author (Elizabeth Lanphier). Hannah's experiences offer possibilities to reimagine concepts of fat and thin in clinical practice, or, in the language of nutrition, "obesity"/being "overweight" compared to "healthy" or "normal" weight. We use the terms "obese," "obesity," "overweight," "healthy," and "normal" to denote their deployment, but do not adopt them ourselves. It is our hope that this case study helps demystify the mechanisms by which pre-established patterns or narratives—received through culture/socialization, personal experience, anecdote, or professional practice—overshadow counter-narratives presented by a fat body in a medical encounter.

Hannah's story helps us frame the body as text read through narratively warped lenses. These lenses are shaped by the human tendency to fill in incomplete stories as part of pattern-seeking behavior, compounded by social and professional bias. Several dominant narratives implicitly run through our readings of fat bodies within the U.S. context. Anti-fat bias is rooted in anti-Black bias and socio-economic bias (Strings, 2019). Anti-fat bias is also connected to narratives of personal choice that dominate much of western health care practice. Logics of choice, as Mol (2008) describes them, focus on personal "health" choices, and fail to appreciate the structural and systemic conditions within which we operate, and the inter-relational practices of care upon which adequate health care depends. Medical practitioners (like many people[1]) deploy stereotypes about fat bodies within logics of choice, according to which fat bodies result from individual moral failings.

Biases and projections onto fat bodies, are, we propose, failures of imagination. As moral and medical communities, we subscribe to engrained narratives, accepting them as true representations of the world, and we fail to imagine them differently. Imaginative resistance is one way to conceptualize narrative bias arising out of tendencies toward pattern recognition. But imaginative resistance also generates a new avenue to critique anti-fat bias. The concept of imaginative resistance invites imagining otherwise, or seeing anew. Reimagination occurs not

DOI: 10.4324/9781003057000-11

only at the individual level, but also, crucially, at a larger social level among those in shared epistemological and social practices.

Fat bodies are overlooked as sites of oppression because the medicalization of fatness is complicit in narratives of individual choice and health that fail to imagine fatness other than as an individual choice or (moral) failure. Understanding anti-fat bias as part of intersectional oppression points us toward critical models for addressing it. Fat acceptance serves as a crucial missing link in anti-oppression training for health care practitioners. To conclude this chapter, we illustrate how tools from narrative practice can transform clinical training by responding to imaginative resistance.

We suggest pedagogical tools that engage narrative methods help impart future clinicians (including medical, nursing, psychotherapy, dietetics, and physical therapy students) with reading techniques useful in the clinical encounter. Training future clinicians is an upstream solution that puts new, more attuned, clinicians in the pipeline. However, situating training within the framework of imaginative resistance addresses the need for transformative experiences to expand outside the realm of medical education, and into the realm of practice.

The weight—socialization and imagination

Weight, as a concept, whether connected to bodies or not, carries negative moral connotations. Weight often means burden[2] ...

I entered the field of nutrition from a place of loving food. I wanted to understand its effects and how it could be used for good. I was a recipient of the Women, Infants and Children nutrition program and National School Lunch Program growing up and felt intimately familiar with the power—and failures—of those programs. I wanted to focus on nutrition policy, believing there must be a way to make healthy, responsibly produced food available to everyone, rather than the Domino's pizza that was the affordable option in my high school.

My grandfather worked as an allied health professional. In retrospect, I see he was very fatphobic. As a teen I recall arguing with him at a family party. I thought his brother (my great-uncle) should eat what he wanted without getting berated by my grandfather and our family. My great-uncle had chronic health issues, and while he likely had a high body mass index or BMI (if I had known at the time how to calculate BMI), he was muscular and active. My intuition was that people should eat what they want, if they can, and it makes them happy. Practices of fat shaming rubbed me the wrong way, yet fatphobia was a core aspect of my socialization. My grandfather saw health as a reward for virtue and self-deprivation. He discussed these attitudes with an almost religious fervor when talking about how he warned his patients of the ills that would befall them if they did not start restricting their food intake and body size.

The first diet I was aware of was the Atkin's diet. My grandmothers dieted on-and-off throughout my early life and dabbled in Weight Watchers. But the Atkins craze was the first time I remember a diet featuring in people's habits and conversations. I lived with one of my grandmothers the summer she was on the Atkins diet. She lost quite a bit of weight; everyone gave her compliments. She went on a victory shopping trip at the only mall around, an hour from home. Her life seemed to be transformed. As a kid I was nicknamed "Chunky Style" by boys in my PE class. Girls from my basketball team laughed in the locker room when my belly hung over my gym shorts. As a pudgy junior high schooler, I wondered: would that one day be me? But I equally recall the pain on my grandmother's face after ultimately gaining back the lost weight, after "letting things slip," as she would say.

My current work and research help me to understand how I was socialized and encultured to believe that "eradicating obesity" was not only reasonable, but righteous. I was trained to enter a patient room with so many preconceptions about "obesity" and "health" that I was being taught to impose onto the clinical encounter.

For Hannah, her family (especially grandparents) and peers reinforced a moral landscape that constructed thinness as a symbol of moral triumph and social value, and fatness as a site of moral failure worthy of public shame and condemnation. Hannah's narrative highlights the importance of understanding the culture of weight stigma and anti-fat bias in the field of nutrition (Jung et al., 2015). Nutrition researchers and clinicians are not only socialized inside fatphobic culture, they also are the custodians of it (Schwartz et al., 2003). Thus, their internalized narratives, fostered by the field of clinical nutrition, also serve to reinforce the authority of anti-fat bias.

My hope in pursing nutrition as a career was to support "good" habits for young people, with the belief this would prevent them from spending their lives chained to dieting. Research showed that "overweight" children became "obese" adults, but I thought that I was living proof that that wasn't necessarily true. I had been an "overweight kid," and I was convinced that my acquired thinness was my "reward" for playing sports, exercising regularly, and eating healthfully at home.

I didn't think everyone had to be thin, but I knew what it felt like to not have thin privilege (a term I only learned years later). I could help young people avoid fatness, to have a "healthy" body, through nutrition. At the time I failed to see how this work was just promoting problematic fatphobia that failed to imagine fat bodies as "healthy." And I did not see how my savior complex and personal narrative contributed to my own imaginative failures.

Much of the research on healthy food access when I entered the field of nutrition was (and remains) centered on "obesity." So, I intended to become an expert in it. I took at face value the rigors of research, and interpreted the abundance of scholarship, funding, and focus on "obesity" within nutrition to be testament to its correctness. Never did I stop to think about what was silent in the conversation. Euphemisms like "obesity" were thrown around to avoid saying the word "fat." And no one ever said "thin," but it was implicit when referencing "normal" or "healthy" weight. It didn't cross my mind that I was joining a crusade for thinness. Similar to how whiteness goes unnamed in discussions of race, thinness was simply taken as the default, the assumed ideal.

Hannah's story shows how she was being trained in a community of practition-ers in which shared practices are expressive of normative, collectively held views and the practices communicate those views. These expressive-communicative practices shape the group as a coherent collective, organized around common views. Feminist philosopher Margaret Urban Walker (2007) describes morality as "woven through the way people live; it both shapes and is shaped by the rules, roles, and assumptions that constitute a social world," such that "moral under-standings will be expressed through social ones," and "social identities and roles will include moral understandings as working parts" (p. ix). In other words, our social realities shape and are shaped by our moral understandings in mutually reflexive ways. This is distinct from the assumption of any kind of fixed morality separate from the social groups that shape and enact it.

Walker's work echoes that of Ludwig Wittgenstein (2009), who conceptu-alizes the ways normative ideas enter into our practices as "language games." He describes that we make meaning of words within a community of language game "players" who conjointly make, reinforce, and codify their meaning. Once these meanings enter into our routine practices, we take for granted that they are constructed definitions: they simply are the way things are. Wittgenstein uncovers the shifting normative aspects of language: he describes language as an ancient city upon which expanding new suburbs can be built outward.

Norms, rules, and codes can be revised, changed, and built upon, both in lan-guage, but more broadly, in ethics and social customs. Social practices also work like language games: we develop them in conversation with our moral community, and then fail to see them as socially constructed practices. For Wittgenstein (2009), lan-guage games are a model for understanding moral norms, in which there is always the possibility to, as he says, "see as" differently, or "see anew." Yet it takes the community of language game players to imagine differently, and to be the vanguard of change involves confronting substantial imaginative resistance, or failures of imagination.

Part of seeing anew requires us to see critically that which has become familiar, internalized, normalized, or unquestioned. Seeing anew is part of the path to social change: once you see differently, you cannot go back to seeing as you did before, because what is "hidden in plain sight" has now been revealed. Yet we don't always look for ways to see what we don't know could be seen differently: this is imaginative resistance. In Hannah's story, various actors don't know to imagine other than valorizing thinness or blaming fatness. And in her nutrition and public health training, she confronts resistance to imagining "obesity" as anything other than a public and personal health problem.

Imaginative resistance

In my training in nutrition and public health, it was a given that "obesity" was a problem. The fields reinforced fatphobia. The majority of lectures start with a familiar set of slides: either a heat map of the globe or a map of the United States appears; the lecturer recounts the gravity of the "obesity epi-demic;" locations on the map get darker and darker in color as residents are designated to have a BMI over 25 kg/m^2. These slides are clicked through hastily, affirming grave and ominous trends that the audience unanimously accepts.

Most of the data presented in nutrition and public health studies was accepted uncritically so long as it supported and justified the mission to "eradicate obesity." Only when data contradicted the accepted knowledge that fatness—"obesity"—was a clinical problem, was it challenged. A prime example is the Flegal et al. (2013) meta-analysis of all-cause mortality and high BMI. The paper reported that having an "overweight" BMI was associated with significantly lower all-cause mortality, and "Grade 1 obesity" was not associated with higher mortality. The paper incited outrage within the fields of public health and nutrition: it implied that being thin wasn't ideal, being fat may not be a problem, and fatness might have significant "health" benefits. This flew in the face of everything we had been trained to believe. Scholars sought to discredit the findings, including challenging the study methodology without acknowledging the same methodological constraints in their own works. I have been assigned this paper in no less than three courses, and in each one the instructor concludes that the paper had to be wrong.

Hannah's narrative highlights the true weight of resistance. She was being trained to see the world of health and nutrition through a particular narrative lens.

In my public health courses, the most common example of a health problem offered in any class, whether about nutrition or not, is "obesity." It's everyone's favorite exposure or outcome.

But if Hannah's education in nutrition, health, and body size, both culturally and formally, is like an ancient city, she then builds out new streets and suburbs of thought, some of which run askew from the pathway she was previously on …

I started to perceive how core elements of our work triggered disordered eating and weight obsession among those of us training to be dietitians and health practitioners. In one course we spent a class measuring each other's body fat percentage using calipers. People openly voiced that they were afraid of "knowing" what the activity would uncover about their health. They made preemptive apologies about why they hadn't been eating well or exercising as much as they "should." The student with the lowest body fat percentage was praised widely at the end of the activity. In retrospect, the lanugo on her arms and temporal wasting were evident signs of malnutrition. In other classes, we were asked to keep food journals and questionnaires. Our food intake was measured and assessed. Each of these activities was meant to strengthen our skills as clinicians and researchers. Yet the emotional and psychic distress it caused us as individuals was palpable. But none of us voiced concern about how these same activities might affect patients or research study participants, even as it caused us anguish.

When I started working with patients, I noticed the unintentional pressures I exerted. I worked in a clinic in Southeastern Michigan, and most of my patients were Black and Brown girls who came to see me for what they thought of as "weight problems."

Identity markers include categories like race, ethnicity, gender, sex, socio-economic status, education, age, all of which may influence body size, while fatness itself can be an intersecting site of oppression. Just as people might be inclined to perform aspects of their identity, either playing up or playing down expected racial, gender, sexual "norms," we might also perform our constructed notions of "health." Hannah's fellow nutrition students performed their own ingrained assumptions about health and body size in the classroom, just as Hannah's patients also performed their concepts of health for her in clinic ...

My teenage patients would wince as they stepped onto the scale in the routine weight check that started our appointments. Patients told me what they thought I wanted to hear and performed their health for me. I became aware of this performance once I saw it start to fall away as I worked more closely with my patients. Once they knew that I wasn't going to chastise them for eating multiple helpings of mac and cheese at a family reunion, they were more likely to report their eating habits beyond simply what they thought I wanted to hear. Usually, initial visits involved details about their attempts to eat vegetables at every meal, or descriptions of consuming only what they believed to be "healthy snacks." In later sessions, patients would admit that they had only eaten those snacks once in their life, or that they couldn't remember the last time they'd eaten a vegetable that wasn't corn.

Over time I realized patient "performance" of perceived "health" was in part because my patients did not anticipate positive experiences with health care providers: they were working to maintain our positive interactions while worrying that it was all conditional. In my training, I was told to never react to a dietary recall because it would make the patient less likely to provide honest responses. In my practice this wasn't hard; I was of the mind that foods were not "good" or "bad." Yet I found that patients would expect praise when reporting perceived "healthy eating." When I did not react, they would try to prompt praise, asking "isn't that good?"

Patients that had expressed a weight loss goal often talked about being terrified to step on a scale. Even those who didn't voice their worry often looked panic-stricken when I suggested we check their weight. A patient once asked if we could do weigh-ins at the end of their visit so that they didn't have to "see the look of disappointment on your face." Any disappointment on my face was empathizing with a patient who had not met their goal, not because of my own expectations for them.

Yet I understood that they perceived the look on my face as indicating they let me down (they had not). I spent hours in my office with sobbing young women, trying to convince them that at the age of 14 years old their body wasn't broken simply because of the number on a scale or their inability to change it.

For Hannah's patients, their socialization was not only that their bodies were broken but that they, the custodian of the broken body, were also broken. These logics are reinforced by the kinds of "language games," or ingrained narratives that equate weight with a "problem," as Hannah describes. Her patients read their own bodies as unruly problems requiring fixing, or at least containment. They also defend themselves against the assumed narrative of their own impurity, performing rites of health as absolution against their shameful, or even immoral, bodies.

> Our grant money in the clinic where I worked depended on several health markers, one of which was decreasing "child obesity." We routinely issued a newsletter highlighting our so-called success stories. Reviewing the putative success stories from before and during my time at the clinic, I found that all of them were either because someone had gone through a growth spurt right after we met them, or they were patients I later realized were actively engaging in eating disorders.
>
> When I documented eating disorders in my patients, almost without fail they went ignored by fellow clinicians. Even if I detailed a patient's self-report of vomiting to lose weight multiple times a week, or that they passed out in gym because they hadn't eaten more than a handful of chips in 48 hours, my fellow clinicians were hesitant to diagnose an eating disorder.

Was it not possible to read patients in fat bodies as having eating disorders, because their disordered eating did not produce the expected narrative of being thin? Were clinicians instead assessing these disordered practices as self-restraint that produced a good "result"? The underlying metanarrative operative in these encounters is dominated by a false equivalency of body size with health, in which thin bodies are necessarily healthy in ways that fat bodies are not, and therefore even harmful practices, when practiced by someone fat, cannot themselves be unhealthy. In this way these girls were being read to exhibit a moral triumph, not an eating disorder.

> I didn't have enough patients of other racial identities to compare the treatment, but it did not surprise me to later uncover research about how underdiagnosed eating disorders are for fat folks, especially Black and Brown youth (Austin et al., 2013; Cachelin et al., 2001; Coffino et al., 2019; Forrest et al., 2017; Kutz et al., 2020; Swanson et al., 2011). I had a patient I saw regularly for a few months, who came into my office exasperated one day. They had just been in to see another clinician in my clinic and felt they hadn't been heard. As I was reviewing some of the goals we had set at the last session, they stopped me and said "Miss Hannah, it really feels like y'all in here want me to be white,[3] and I'm just never going to be white." This statement struck me both for how pithily this middle schooler had encapsulated the tension I often felt in clinical practice and also how much it resonated with me. I am white coded in most spaces,[4] but I self-identify as Black. The idea of feeling like people wanted me to be white was something I had experienced often

in my life. I had often associated the feeling with the fact that I didn't fit neatly into racial categories. But in this moment with my patient, I realized this was a pressure felt regardless of proximity to whiteness. I also recognized that when my patient said they would never be white, they were not just talking about the fact of their skin color, but also the concept of what is "normal." whiteness is both explicitly in media, and implicitly in much of US society, connected to normalcy, as is being middle class, cisgender, heterosexual, or male.

The narrative expectations of Black and Brown bodies defy assumptions by health care providers regarding received narratives regarding "health," "ideal" body size, and race. Hannah's patient understands, possibly much better than the practitioners supposed to be "caring" for them, that they are held against an idealized body type that is not only a size or shape they will never be, but also a race and color that they will never be. Hannah's experience with this patient illustrates the reflexivity of the clinical encounter: both parties are co-constructing each other and themselves. Rita Charon (2006) writes that "it is in meeting with other selves that the self comes alive" (p. 51). This clinical encounter helps Hannah acknowledge not only the narratively warped lenses through which clinicians often regard their patients, but also the narratively warped lenses with which she is also seen—including by herself, feeling pressure to perform norms of thinness or whiteness that she earlier noted are the social, but also professional, ideals that go unnamed. Not only are patients' bodies expected to adhere to a script of thinness, this script implicitly casts a white body in the role of thin body.

In Hannah's encounter with her patient, we witness how perceptions of thinness and fatness are inextricably racialized. Anti-fat bias and anti-Black bias are intersecting forms of oppression, but also, are mutually producing forms of oppression. Sabrina Strings (2019) has shown that concepts of fatness and thinness were constructed in order to produce, and sustain, white supremacists and anti-Black narratives attributing whiteness with thinness and superiority, and Blackness with fatness and inferiority. Kimberlé Crenshaw's (1989) concept of intersectionality points to how we are not only one identity, but that various aspects of our identity intersect in unique, and at times multiply oppressing ways. For example, as Crenshaw revealed, workplace discrimination lawsuits based only on race or only on gender failed Black women who were multiply oppressed by their race and their gender. Crenshaw (1989, 1990) coined the term intersectionality to describe the layered forms of oppression created by multiple, intersecting identity markers.

Our identity-markers tend to accompany us as facts of our being. While some identity markers are intrinsic, whether or how features of our identity are noticed, and whether or how they privilege or oppress us, are extrinsic. The social and political contexts in which we exist create narrative content that shapes how we come to recognize and evaluate various identity markers. Moreover, some identity markers necessarily change across a lifespan (like age), while others *may* change over time (religious affiliation, socioeconomic status, education). But for the young people, many of whom were Black and Brown girls, comprising Hannah's primary patient population, growing up within social narratives telling them their race, body size, gender, or socioeconomic status are all wrong, they might feel that their weight is one identity marker they can take control of, that they can *make* change. But what Strings' research and Hannah's patient both make clear is that fatness and Blackness (or Brownness) are not only intersecting forms of oppression, but also they are an intermixed oppression: anti-fatness and anti-Blackness feed each other, thin privilege and white privilege mutually benefit each other—unless we imagine otherwise.

Narrative method and transformative pedagogy

Part of what we have thus far suggested is that these biases (against body size and race) are part of socially produced narratives. And while we (as members of moral, social, political, or clinical communities) encounter significant resistance to imagining new narratives, understanding the problem as partially one of imaginative resistance opens channels for recognizing narratives, identifying areas of imaginative resistance, and shaping new narrative pathways that move out from under the weight of this imaginative resistance, failure, and ongoing oppression.

Because fatphobia stems, at least in part, from notions of supremacy historically rooted in anti-Blackness, to truly address inequities in health care and, ultimately, health outcomes, any program of anti-oppression training must recognize the interlocking nature of systems of oppression including racial bias and fat bias. Understanding fat bias as both revealing various intersecting oppressive narratives and concealing the mechanics of such oppression through the practice of imaginative resistance, is instructive to understand anti-fat-bias as part of an intersectional view of oppression in which various identity markers intersect to multiply oppress individuals and groups.

> Biases against fat people shows through in many ways. Whether it's a venerated academic referring to "good people who take care of themselves" when discussing a weight loss intervention, or the victim-blaming present in most "obesity epidemiology" courses. After years of taking that framing at face value, I started to finally understand why those statements made me uncomfortable. It took nearly a decade of actively participating in the field before I knew how to vocalize my discomfort. I had come into the field a skeptic, yet it still took nearly a decade for me to realize how problematic the field of nutrition, and work that I actively engaged in, can be. It concerns me that on my journey toward recognizing nutrition's failures, I likely hurt my own patients along the way. What could it look like for clinicians to come to this realization without propagating and perpetuating undue harm?

This haunting question moves us to consider techniques from narrative practice to transform health care pedagogies across clinical training programs. Though we have analyzed the issue through the field of nutrition, our analysis is not unique to nutrition. Students across clinical practices are all being trained within narratively warped lenses of anti-fatness and can benefit from pedagogies for narrative transformation. Narrative and transformative work is not only part of de-biasing clinical training, practice, and encounters. It is also part of broader anti-oppression training that understands fat bias within an intersectional framework. Narrative tools have continued to be honed and studied in medical practice largely since Charon coined the term "narrative medicine," and offered her conceptual mapping of the goals and process of narrative practice within medicine. The principles of narrative practice in medicine, as proposed by Charon (2001, 2006), are those of attention, representation, and affiliation.

"Attention" means that the medical practitioner directs her attention to her patient's story, to attune to and receive it. "Representation" is not merely the witnessing of a patient's story at work, but is the active engagement with the story, in which the practitioner represents it for herself and also back to the patient, co-constructing the story between the teller and the listener. "Representation" occurs through the active listening of "attention" rather than a passive listening.

Attention and representation, when fully realized, achieve "affiliation" between the practitioner and her patient. This affiliation is a form of cohesion that builds trust, collaboration, and contribution toward a shared goal. In the setting of a clinical encounter between a physician and patient, this goal might be to support a shared view of the patient's health. While patient and practitioner might enter the encounter with prior received narratives of what "health" means and what kinds of bodies are "healthy," narrative methods invite the interrogation and discussion of these constructs, and in ideal circumstances, a shared definition that the patient and practitioner co-construct for the particular patient and her uniquely intersecting circumstances.

In medical education, narrative tools and narrative medicine techniques are gaining growing use to foster empathy and understanding between practitioners and their patients. One study of the impact of narrative teaching during medical school on participant's experiences in their residencies suggested a correlation between narrative medicine training and improved resiliency (Arntfield et al., 2013). The study participants completed was a 1-month course in narrative medicine in which students met weekly during the month to discuss assigned texts, apply close-reading methods, and engage in reflective writing exercises. Participants "expressed that the process of training in narrative medicine was enjoyable and that the outcome was transformative" (p. 282). The study subjects identified narrative methods as building their communication skills, and helping them to better listen for, and empathize with, patient experiences. They also identified the reflective writing practices as fostering skills for personal resilience and better peer understanding and support.

When learning to close read narratives, whether as a literature student, or a medical student, and whether the narrative is a novel by Chimamanda Ngozi Adichie or a patient story in clinic, narrative analysis trains attention on the mechanics of the narrative itself: tone, tense, narrator, time, setting, language, dialect, etc. Some stories become so familiar to us that we assume they just are:

Romeo and Juliet are star-crossed lovers, Julius Cesar was honorable, and King Lear tragic.[5] The stories become expected, received, and unquestioned. Yet these and other texts continue to be sites of reflection and study because close reading, especially within evolving social and political contexts, brings new information to the stories and identifies new narrative interpretations or applications of even the most classic texts.

Similarly, close reading patients (their stories and their bodies) with attention to narrative details challenges imaginative resistance by inviting the possibility for a novel reading or a new interpretation of what would otherwise be expected, received, or presumed. Narrative methods in medical education are one piece then of challenging imaginative resistance specifically with regards to fat bodies and constructing new (counter) narratives within medical communities, and between patients and practitioners.

Narrative techniques to address imaginative resistance ought to be understood, however, as part of a larger project of transformative pedagogy situated within the broader rubric of anti-oppression education and intervention for medical trainees. As we have suggested, to understand anti-fat-bias as only a problem of body size discrimination, without connecting it to a history of racialized oppression against Black and Brown bodies is its own imaginative failure.

Hannah's experience of imagining anew has led her to re-imagine classroom practices with her own students:

> As teachers-in-training, my colleagues and I who are concerned about reifying fatphobia set boundaries around using "obesity" as an example. My own students know that when I ask for an example in class of a health "problem," it can't be "obesity." Students will occasionally try to circumvent this boundary by suggesting a measure, such as high BMI or % body fat. Students are culturally programmed to see "obesity" as the health problem par excellence, as though weight and fatness stand in for markers of poor health.

Hannah challenges the imaginative resistance she encounters among her students, and invites them to narrate different stories about health, fatness, and weight. The work of generating new narratives and actively re-imagining concepts of weight and health contribute to at least two projects.

One project, when thinking about training students entering into clinical practice, is to build capacities for attention, representation, and affiliation internal to clinical encounters. That is to say, to better attend to patients, represent their concerns, needs, and realities, and affiliate with them around shared goals of health and care that are co-constructed.

The other project takes up attention, representation, and affiliation in the aggregate, as we shape our moral communities in which we, as Walker (2007) suggests, express and communicate our shared values and practices. And rather than moralizing weight and fatness within medicine as moral failing, narrative practice affords us an opportunity to confront our imaginative failings, and to imagine anew in affiliation with others and our intersectional differences.

Notes

1 We are not suggesting this is unique to medical practice, only that it has unique repercussions within medical practice.
2 Thank you to Leah Lomotey-Nakon for being a conversation partner as we worked on this project, and for pointing out this particular connection.
3 In this text, the word "white" is not capitalized due to the long history of hate groups capitalizing it to further reinforce socially constructed hierarchy and validate notions of supremacy. I use "white" here to refer to skin tone vs. "Black," which refers to a people with a common set of experiences through shared culture and history.
4 Being "white coded" here means "viewed as white" by others. Similar to the notion of "street race," this is the racial categorization assigned by others, based predominantly on race-associated physical features. For Hannah: *when strangers see me, they assume I am white and treat me as such. This term is used to distinguish from the notion of "passing as white," which historically implies intent and actively engaging systems of anti-Blackness to gain privileges and advantages. While I identify as Black and make no secret of it, I recognize that I receive white privilege through this social coding and do not experience the same level of anti-Black racism that my family members who are coded as Black experience.* (For further discussion of racial coding and street race, see López et al., 2018 and Vowel, 2017.)
5 A set of examples from Shakespeare already selects a type of narrative expectation that these will be culturally familiar and relevant, and perhaps risks further centering a particular kind of Western, white, male canon. Yet this in part furthers the point about narrative patterns and dominance.

References

Arntfield, S. L., Slesar, K., Dickson, J., & Charon, R. (2013). Narrative medicine as a means of training medical students toward residency competencies. *Patient Education and Counseling, 91*(3), 280–286. https://doi.org/10.1016/j.pec.2013.01.014

Austin, S. B., Nelson, L. A., Birkett, M. A., Calzo, J. P., & Everett, B. (2013). Eating disorder symptoms and obesity at the intersections of gender, ethnicity, and sexual orientation in US high school students. *American Journal of Public Health, 103*(2), e16–e22. https://doi.org/10.2105/AJPH.2012.301150

Cachelin, F. M., Rebeck, R., Veisel, C., & Striegel-Moore, R. H. (2001). Barriers to treatment for eating disorders among ethnically diverse women. *International Journal of Eating Disorders, 30*(3), 269–278. https://doi.org/10.1002/eat.1084

Charon, R. (2001). Narrative medicine: A model for empathy, reflection, profession, and trust. *Journal of the American Medical Association, 286*(15), 1897–1902. https://doi.org/10.1001/jama.286.15.1897

Charon, R. (2006). *Narrative medicine: Honoring the stories of illness.* Oxford University Press.

Coffino, J. A., Udo, T., & Grilo, C. M. (2019). Rates of help-seeking in US adults with lifetime DSM-5 eating disorders: Prevalence across diagnoses and differences by sex and ethnicity/race. *Mayo Clinic Proceedings, 94*(8), 1415–1426. https://doi.org/10.1016/j.mayocp.2019.02.030

Crenshaw, K. (1989). Demarginalizing the intersection of race and sex: A Black feminist critique of antidiscrimination doctrine, feminist theory and antiracist politics. *University of Chicago Legal Forum, 140*, 139–167.

Crenshaw, K. (1990). Mapping the margins: Intersectionality, identity politics, and violence against women of color. *Stanford Law Review, 43*, 1241–1299. https://doi.org/10.2307/1229039

Flegal, K. M., Kit, B. K., Orpana, H., & Graubard, B. I. (2013). Association of all-cause mortality with overweight and obesity using standard body mass index categories: A systematic review and meta-analysis. *Journal of the American Medical Association, 309*(1), 71–82. https://doi.org.10.1001/jama.2012.113905

Forrest, L. N., Smith, A. R., & Swanson, S. A. (2017). Characteristics of seeking treatment among US adolescents with eating disorders. *International Journal of Eating Disorders, 50*(7), 826–833. https://doi.org/10.1002/eat.22702

Jung, F. U., Luck-Sikorski, C., Wiemers, N., & Riedel-Heller, S. G. (2015). Dietitians and nutritionists: Stigma in the context of obesity. A systematic review. *PloS One, 10*(10), e0140276. https://doi.org/10.1371/journal.pone.0140276

Kutz, A. M., Marsh, A. G., Gunderson, C. G., Maguen, S., & Masheb, R. M. (2020). Eating disorder screening: A systematic review and meta-analysis of diagnostic test characteristics of the SCOFF. *Journal of General Internal Medicine, 35*(3), 885–893. https://doi.org/10.1007/s11606-019-05478-6

López, N., Vargas, E., Juarez, M., Cacari-Stone, L., & Bettez, S. (2018). What's your "street race"? Leveraging multidimensional measures of race and intersectionality for examining physical and mental health status among Latinxs. *Sociology of Race and Ethnicity, 4*(1), 49–66. https://doi.org/10.1177/2332649217708798

Mol, A. (2008). *The logic of care: Health and the problem of patient choice.* Routledge.

Schwartz, M. B., Chambliss, H. O. N., Brownell, K. D., Blair, S. N., & Billington, C. (2003). Weight bias among health professionals specializing in obesity. *Obesity Research, 11*(9), 1033–1039. https://doi.org/10.1038/oby.2003.142

Strings, S. (2019). *Fearing the Black body: The racial origins of fat phobia.* New York University Press.

Swanson, S. A., Crow, S. J., Le Grange, D., Swendsen, J., & Merikangas, K. R. (2011). Prevalence and correlates of eating disorders in adolescents: Results from the national comorbidity survey replication adolescent supplement. *Archives of General Psychiatry, 68*(7), 714–723. https://doi.org/10.1001/archgenpsychiatry.2011.22

Vowel, C. [@apihtawikosisan]. (2017, March 23). "'White coded' Indigenous ppl and settler colonialism" thread [Tweet]. Twitter. https://twitter.com/i/events/844936637754884096

Walker, M. U. (2007). *Moral understandings: A feminist study in ethics.* Oxford University Press.

Wittgenstein, L. (2009). *Philosophical investigations* (rev. 4th ed.). (G.E.M. Anscombe, P.M.S. Hacker, & J. Schulte, Trans). Wiley-Blackwell.

10 What counts as good or bad writing about weight

Reflections of a writing coach

Heather A. Brown

I'm just going to say it: the vast majority of medical and science writers are not great compositionists. This is not a new sentiment, by any means. Heath (2018) argued that most scientific or medical writing was grounded in jargon and incomprehensible in structure. Radovsky (1979) complained articles in medical journals were hard to understand, making them nearly useless for a medical doctor like him to use in his work. Before that, Gregg (1957) found that the "… common level of medical and scientific writing in our professional books and journals constitutes the most serious internal limitation to medical education and research" (p. 58). And, in 1900, the editors of the *Journal of the American Medical Association* (1900) also complained about the fact that medical scholars cannot write.

If medical writing in general is less than stellar, individuals who write about weight issues tend to be downright awful. As a set of general observations from my years of experience in the field, over and over again I have seen poorly sourced literature reviews with no critical engagement with the literature, confirmation bias, oversimplification of complex medical issues, assumptions about the intelligence and behavior of fat people, lack of data for a variety of assertions about the connection between weight and health, and an inability to delineate between correlation and causation.

As someone who loves words and communication, I find the language used in many written pieces about fat individuals to be particularly egregious. First, there is the language of suffering. In the pieces I review for authors, fat people suffer so much that life must hardly be worth living. In addition, fat people are not human. They are people with "obesity," as if somehow fat individuals do not inhabit their own bodies but are some sort of a larvae just waiting for their adipose tissue to melt away so they can become human. And then, there are the millions of bad puns and hyperbole. I would blame Morgan Spurlock (2004) and his smirk from *Super Size Me,* but the puns and value-laden statements started long before he came on the scene. For example, DeAngelis (as cited in Sargent & Blanchflower, 1994, p. 681) wrote:

> It seems that it's over for the "fat lady" long before she sings. Obese teenage girls can look forward to a double whammy in earning power because of two physical features, size and gender. Does anyone doubt that the same is true in America?

DOI: 10.4324/9781003057000-12

On the other hand, Kobayashi (2009) takes his words straight from Spurlock, when he observes that, "It is very common these days to encounter 'super-sized' students on the campuses of many colleges and universities in the USA" (p. 555), while Singh and McMahan (2006) ratchet the hyperbole up by arguing that fat tissue is as dangerous as "the threats of bio-terrorism and small pox" (p. 207). I have even worked on a grant proposal for a tenured faculty member who wrote, "Diabetes mellitus and obesity have reached global pandemic proportions, rivaling the combined morbidity and mortality of the Black Death plague and influenza epidemics."

As a writing coach, academic editor, grant editor, and editor of a peer-reviewed journal, my mission is to help individuals write clearly and concisely about complex topics and learn how to better communicate scientific information that can be used to design and implement unbiased, evidence-based policy and practice. Currently, the writing I see from individuals writing about fat people does not come close to that ideal. This chapter presents some of the challenges I see in academic writing about fatness and presents alternatives that will not only strengthen the writing abilities of individuals writing about fat people but also help them in a way that will not further stigmatize or harm the individuals about whom they write.

Good writing about weight

If medical and scientific writing is generally poor and writing on fat individuals is specifically problematic, what constitutes good medical and scientific writing about fat people? Many guides to writing for scientists and medical professionals focus on what I consider the nuts and bolts of writing: spelling, grammar, sentence construction, avoidance of jargon, using active as opposed to passive voice, and the like (see Garrett, 2017, as an example). Some more advanced tips for good writing include a focus on writing good paragraphs, where each paragraph centers on a singular core idea, and using clear and concise sentences (Savage & Yeh, 2019). Authors are urged to review and revise their writing and to seek outside readers to provide feedback and guidance. The tools of the trade are featured extensively, and writers are often told or shown how to use LaTeX (a document preparation software used by many in the scientific and technical fields), various citation generators, and reference trackers. Finally, there is a focus on publishing—how to find a journal, how to write a cover letter, and how to prepare a manuscript for submission (Garrett, 2017; Savage & Yeh, 2019).

Writing about weight and the lives of fat individuals requires more than this or medical and science writing will continue to portray fat individuals as data points, cautionary tales, or non-sentient flesh cocoons that must be changed and manipulated. There is a better way.

Fat Studies is a discipline that approaches "the construction of fat and fatness with a critical methodology—the same sort of progressive, systematic academic rigor with which we approach negative attitudes and stereotypes about women, queer people, and racial groups" (Solovay & Rothblum, 2009, p. 2). As a general rule, Fat Studies focuses on the actual lived experiences of fat individuals as fat indi-viduals understand their own experiences. This is an especially important point to consider when writing about fatness, since "obesity" rhetoric, which dominates medical and scientific research and writing about fatness, tends to portray fat people as "…abstracted and largely absent from the discourse …" (Cooper, 2010, p. 1023).

There are four critical characteristics of Fat Studies as a theoretical framework (Brown, 2012, 2016, 2017). The first is that the framework actively challenges bias and discrimination against fat individuals. This activist focus also means that Fat Studies problematizes the dominant "obesity" discourse that uncritically medi-calizes fat individuals as diseased, the second main characteristic of Fat Studies. Third, Fat Studies calls for the actual lived experiences of fat individuals to be placed at the center of research, writing, policy, and practice whenever weight issues are involved in research, writing, policy, and practice. Finally, language about fatness and how language is used to talk about fatness must be considered in all medical and scientific writing about fatness. Each of these four components can be applied to medical and scientific writing about weight in such a way as to create good writing that is grounded in genuine care, considers the needs and wants of fat individuals as living human beings, and presents data in a way that avoids further stigmatizing or harming a stigmatized population.

A note of clarification

I must begin with my own clarification. This chapter is not about my current job. I have had a career as a professional writer and academic editor, in one genre or another, for over 20 years. The areas I focus on here are problematic areas not only for undergraduate and graduate students across many disciplines but also for journalists, researchers, faculty, and health care providers. The examples come from papers, grant applications, and other forms of written communication that I have worked with a regular basis over the last decade.

Common issues found in problematic writing on weight

In this section, I will focus on three major areas where I commonly see issues that are problematic in medical and scientific writing about fat individuals: sourcing, language, and content. Whenever possible, I will present an example or examples of the area of concern, an analysis of why it is problematic, and discuss how it might be reworked or reframed in order to avoid contributing to further bias and dis-crimination aimed at fat individuals. In all cases, any details that might be used to identify either individuals or their institutions have been removed or anonymized.

Sources

A critically important step in any form of academic writing is a review of the liter-ature. What is already known about a topic? Where are the data published? How rigorous is the methodology that contributed to the collection of the data? How were the data analyzed? What's missing? What is still not known? Are there alternative explanations for the data that have not been considered in the literature?

Unfortunately, many of the papers and grants I review run into challenges at this stage. Often the issue is that the document in question does not allow for an exhaustive literature review. As a result, the material tends to be superficial, mostly a quick summary of a few articles with which the writer engaged. In some cases, the author has not done more than reviewed the abstract of the paper they include in their literature review. In other, more extensive literature reviews, however, writers can still run into concerns if they do not fully vet their sources. Is that journal peer reviewed? How reputable is the journal? How rigorous is the peer review process of the journal? Has the article been corrected or retracted?

Using sources retracted due to misconduct

Retraction of research publications is not uncommon, especially in the medical or hard sciences. Sometimes, it is a matter of other researchers not being able to replicate results. It happens and is an important part of the scientific process. Other times published manuscripts are retracted due to research fraud or misconduct. Fanelli (2009) found that at least 34% of scientists admitted they had engaged or would engage in problematic research practices such as data picking while 2% admitted they had falsified their research—often in pursuit of prestige, tenure, or research funding.

Those who write about weight need to be especially careful to fully vet any resource they use. There is a significant amount of research funding available for issues that deal with weight and health, and this may drive research misconduct. For example, in fiscal year 2019, the National Institutes of Health (2020) alone invested approximately $289 million to combat childhood "obesity" and just over a billion dollars to combat adult "obesity." The competition is fierce for this research funding and the prestige that it imparts which can contribute to a climate that facilitates and rewards cheating and misconduct, particularly in the biomedical research fields (Alberts et al., 2014; Anderson et al., 2007; Casadevall & Fang, 2012; Davis et al., 2007; Stephan, 2012; Teitelbaum, 2008).

Two sources I see used frequently fall into this area of concern. The first are works by Brian Wansink, former Cornell University professor and director of the Food and Brand Lab. Wansink published hundreds of peer-reviewed articles over the course of his career, all of them focused on promoting healthy eating behaviors; his research impacted food policy in the United States at the highest levels (Hamblin, 2018). After an investigation by Cornell, Wansink was found guilty of research misconduct that included "misreporting of research data, problematic statistical techniques, failure to properly document and preserve research results, and inappropriate authorship" (Kotlikoff, 2018, para. 2). Wansink resigned, and more than a dozen of his papers were retracted (Hamblin, 2018).

The second problematic sources I see often are works by former Harvard Medical School Assistant Professor Robert B. Fogel. Fogel was the researcher and author behind a study "proving" a connection between obstructive sleep apnea and "obesity" (see Fogel et al., 2003). In 2009, Fogel was found to have falsified the data for his study so that his data would support his hypothesis (U.S. Department of Health and Human Services, 2009).

These cases are highly problematic because their work served as a foundation for other studies that may contribute to the pathologizing of fatness and present fat individuals as diseased and needing to be cured. Moreover, although the retracted works are noted as such, not all medical or science writers, especially beginning writers, are sufficiently diligent about vetting sources. For example, although the editors of *SLEEP* very clearly state that neither Fogel et al. (2003) nor its preliminary abstract should be referenced or cited, it still finds its way into pieces I review. Given that a fictitious article has been cited over 400 times (Harzing & Kroonenberg, 2017), it is disappointing but not surprising that retracted sources still find their way into documents. Good writing about fatness will use only reputable sources, will be extra diligent about uncovering and avoiding using data by researchers implicated in research misconduct, and remain appropriately skeptical about the validity of any publication that has in its lineage a foundational source that has been flagged or retracted due to research misconduct.

Confirmation bias in selecting sources

An author in a document I have reviewed writes in their introduction:

Obesity is a national epidemic in the United States and is becoming an increasing health problem worldwide. Obesity affects a person's health in many ways and puts both children and adults at greater risk of having chronic illnesses (Mitchell, Catenacci, Wyatt, & Hill, 2011).[1] Obesity has been directly linked to coronary disease, diabetes 2, cancer, sleep apnea, hypertension, osteoarthritis, depression, and liver and gallbladder diseases (Akil & Ahmad, 2011). Risk factors for cardiovascular disease are accentuated when obesity is added to a list of comorbidities. Excess weight increases blood pressure, lipids, and glucose; leading to hypertension, high cholesterol, and diabetes 2; all will directly affect the cardiovascular system (Akil & Ahmad, 2011). The effects of obesity are even worse when the patient is a young child. Children will develop the same risk factors and diseases but sooner in life, which makes long-term health poor. Children are having increased incidence of diabetes 2, fatty liver disease, metabolic syndrome, and joint problems, related to obesity. (Abrams, Katz, & Lorraine, 2011)

Overall, this paragraph is not irredeemable. It has some basic problems—some awkward sentences, grammatical errors, and incorrect terminology; it doesn't flow as well as it could and has too many topics for a single paragraph. The major issue, here, however, is that this paragraph was it. There was no further analysis of the source manuscripts. The writer did not explore the studies, did not analyze the rigor of the research methodology, and did not provide any specific data points that support the assertions made in their writing. In other words, it appears that they looked for and used only those sources that supported the point they wanted to make. The writer of the example engaged in confirmation bias.

I have found that confirmation bias is a major flaw in many medical and scientific pieces on fatness (Brown, 2012). For example, in my own research on the interactions of weight, gender, and learning, I have found that the peer-reviewed published manuscripts I explore as part of my literature reviews are nearly always framed by an introduction and a conclusion that assumes that poor academic performance is correlated with fatness. The authors of these published works do not engage in any analysis of what has come before; rather, they only summarize those previous pieces of literature that confirm their assumptions.

Good writing about weight and fatness needs to do more than summarize previous literature, especially when that literature reinforces the concept of fatness as disease. Good writing will engage with disconfirming evidence rather than accepting previous research at face value. Such an exercise will allow the good writer to not only identify potential pitfalls—including using problematic or retracted literature—but also identify any counter arguments to their own thesis, thereby making their piece more complete and far stronger than a simple rehash.

Language and word choice

Once sources have been identified, vetted, and analyzed for strength and weakness, then the actual process of writing can begin. Writing, at its core, is a form of communication, and the words and phrases selected can help or hinder communication. Good writing about fatness requires a more intense engagement with writing than other types of medical or scientific writing because poor writing about fatness risks creating future harm to fat individuals.

Puns

"Can I use this word here? Or is there another, more appropriate term? I want to be sensitive in my word choices, but I also want to suggest a, well, well-roundedness to this concern." A doctoral student with whom I have been working for a couple of years wants to discuss word choice in her opening paragraph. She has proposed writing that "'obesity' is a well-rounded disorder that may affect the cardiopulmonary system" but she is also conscientious. We have discussed issues of bias and discrimination, and she does not wish to contribute to the trend. She is worried that the term *well-rounded* may be considered a rude pun. I agree with her that her concerns are valid, but also suggest that the word does not convey her actual meaning. She actually wants to write about "obesity" as complex in terms of its relationship with the health of the heart and lungs. After discussion, she decides that she actually needs to rework her opening, add citations instead of making blanket assertions of fact that may be challenged by critical "obesity" researchers engaging with her work, and reframe her thesis so that she is focusing on the health issue—cardiovascular disease—and how a physical therapist might contribute to preventing heart disease through their practice—regardless of a patient's weight.

Avoiding ill-chosen and potentially discriminatory words is important when writing about fat individuals. A few readers may get a little chuckle out of reading some ill-written pun about fat people, but the presence of that pun erases the humanity of a fat person and makes them, a member of an already stigmatized population, the further target of bad jokes. For example, Vastag (2004), no doubt, thought the title "Obesity Is Now on Everyone's Plate" was quite cunning, but its clever implication tying weight to eating is both cruel and incorrect and also obfuscates the actual content of his piece.

Avoiding the language of suffering also is important. In most writing I review that focuses on "obesity" as a disease state, the authors write that fat individuals "suffer from obesity." This wording makes sense in a framework that medicalizes fatness as a disease instead of simply another state of being. In the dominant "obesity" framework, "obese" people are, indeed, suffering, and weight is an illness that must be eradicated for the fat person's own good. This is inaccurate, and the situation is far more complex than that. Some fat people do indeed suffer from their weight, but many other fat individuals only suffer because they are subjected to bias, discrimination, and stigma. However, in much of the writing I review, it is not enough that fat individuals suffer from "obesity." Rather, they suffer from all manner of other things that may or may not be related to the size of their body. For example, one public health student trying to develop a community anti-"obesity" intervention program writes that "the … family is currently disengaged from their community and also suffer from 'obesity.'" My pushback here is that the writer needs to explain how those things are connected and prove the connection.

Person-first language?

Another language construction that I see in medical and scientific writing about fatness is person-first language. Fat people are never fat people; they are people with fat or people with "obesity." This is a result of a major push by medical researchers and practitioners to use this type of language as a way to avoid or eliminate bias. According to the Obesity Action Coalition (n.d.), the following anti-"obesity" organizations have all officially adopted person-first language: American Society for Metabolic and Bariatric Surgery, The Obesity Society, Obesity Medicine Association, Academy of Nutrition and Dietetics, American Academy of Orthopaedic Surgeons, World Obesity Federation, College of Contemporary Health, International Federation for the Surgery of Obesity and Metabolic Disorders, European Association for the Study of Obesity, and the European Coalition for People Living with Obesity.

Kyle and Puhl (2014) argue that "[u]sing stigmatizing language to describe people with 'obesity' or referring to them as 'the obese' can contribute to the already pervasive weight bias present in health care settings" (p. 1211). Palad and Stanford (2018) even took colleagues to task in an editorial when their piece in *The American Journal of Clinical Nutrition* used the phrase "obese people" in a manuscript. According to Kyle and Puhl (2014), using person-first language when writing about or referring to fat individuals is less stigmatizing than the alternatives.

They argue that "[o]bese is an identity. 'Obesity' is a disease. By addressing the disease separately from the person—and doing it consistently—we can pursue this disease while fully respecting the people affected" (Kyle & Puhl, 2014, p. 1211). In other words, hate and destroy the sin while loving and saving the sinners.

At this point word choice becomes tricky for medical and scientific writers writing about fat people. Not everyone agrees that using person-first language is less stigmatizing. Dennett (n.d.) argues that person-first language still carries stigma since it is only used in conjunction with language that is attached to a "negative" condition in the first place. "For example, many say 'she's a dietitian' or 'he's Canadian.' They don't say 'she's a person who works in dietetics' or 'he's a person from Canada.'" (Dennett, n.d., para. 3).

There also remains the issue that the words "overweight" and "obese" are value laden as well. Harjunen (2009) argues that a word like "overweight" can never be value neutral in any usage since it is grounded in a norm that positions being over a specific weight as "defective and abnormal (usually in the medical sense)" (p. 21). Words like "obese" and "obesity" are similarly problematic because they identify a size and shape of body as medicalized (Cooper, 1998).

Writers who use a Fat Studies framework, however, argue for the use of words that ought to be value-neutral adjectives, such as "fat," as opposed to medicalized terms. "Currently, in mainstream U.S. society, the O-words, 'overwight' and 'obese,' are considered more acceptable, even more polite, than the F-word, 'fat.' In the field of Fat Studies, there is agreement that the O-words are neither neutral nor benign" (Wann, 2009, p. xii).

What is a writer to do, then? In some cases, the writer may have little to no choice about the language they use. Certainly, I have worked with community-based nonprofits who are writing grants that absolutely must use anti-"obesity" language if they have any hope of being funded. In those cases, the organizations are generally trying to take advantage of a funding system that rewards anti-"obesity" efforts even when the actual work being proposed follows other guidelines, such as those of Health at Every Size (HAES™). In the end, even with potentially problematic language, the programs have been designed in such a way as to prevent or greatly lessen the likelihood of further bias and discrimination against fat individuals. And that is the key when writing about fat individuals and choosing language. Are you simply engaging in semantic word games? Are other aspects of your piece grounded in anti-bias and anti-discrimination efforts? If you are doing research with actual people, have you asked them how they would like to be defined or described? If you use specific words, have you engaged in describing how those specific terms are defined and how they may be a limitation in your work? How have you grounded your work in context?

Content

Writers working in areas touching on weight also need to be conscious of the content of their writing. By content, I do not mean their literature reviews or even reporting their results, if they are writing about their own research efforts. Rather,

I am suggesting that writers need to focus on avoiding biased and discriminatory content that will be used to influence policy, legislation, and practice, content that—if not presented in a nuanced and careful manner—could become harmful. Specifically, I often see content that does not differentiate between correlation and causation, that oversimplifies a highly complex issue that is not settled science by any means, that makes a number of assertions of facts about the connections between weight and health that are not supported by evidence, or that include problematic assumptions about the intelligence and behavior of fat individuals.

For example, take the following piece. The writer is looking at barriers faced by individuals who wish to lose weight. One barrier the writer describes is the body acceptance movement. They write:

> Currently there is a culture of acceptance for all body sizes and being 'obese' has become normalized, leading some to believe that they can be 'obese' and healthy (Singleton, 2020). Lin and McFerran (2016) found that this acceptance led to more unhealthy behaviors such as eating more and decreasing activity. Glorifying 'overweight' and 'obese' celebrities makes it socially acceptable to be obese and lowers the motivation for people to lose weight. (Lin & McFerran, 2016; Singleton, 2020)

The issue with this content is that it does not provide any definitions for what is meant by body acceptance. It provides a single source for the argument that being "obese" is normalized. It ignores research around the "obesity" paradox and makes assumptions about the connections between body size and health, without ever defining what it means to be healthy.

In another example, the writer is developing an anti-"obesity" public health intervention. In her proposal, she describes individuals in a neighborhood as "suffering from obesity," and suggests, without any data or any citations, that they are "obese" because they are lazy and lack motivation. Part of her program involves identifying individuals who are new to the neighborhood who can model good behavior for the "obese" people already living there. The program suggests that the new neighbors invite the fat neighbors over for dinner so that they can "be educated on preparing healthy meals and also on portion controls, which require one to have control over one's actions but also believing that one is capable of executing self-control actions." Such a program would also serve as an immediate form of portion control since the fat families would be "out of their comfort zone, … [and would be] more likely to eat less due to the embarrassment of having to ask for seconds."

In a final example, a physical therapist writes that—in order to eradicate "obesity"—fat people must "increase fruits and vegetables and decrease fats and carbohydrates in one's daily diet." He argues, without citation, that there are numerous policies and programs to help "low socioeconomic and minority populations" acquire and eat healthy foods, and yet they "all still remain obese." He proposes that individuals who receive food from a food bank or similar program only be allowed to eat fruits and vegetables until they obtain a "healthy weight."

Good writing about weight requires avoiding the fatal flaws demonstrated by the examples above. The connections between weight and health are complex, to say the least, and the connections may be corollary or causal. The writer needs to be able to clearly identify and differentiate between the two. They need to present a more complex picture of how weight may or may not affect health, particularly when issues related to socioeconomic status, access to health care, lack of health insurance, race, gender, sexuality, and other contextual identifiers are in play. Moreover, writers must not make assumptions about the behaviors or intelligence of fat individuals. Assuming that fat people are lazy, unmotivated, make poor choices due to unspecified reasons, or are ignorant about food only stigmatizes them further—and are flat out wrong.

Good intentions, problematic consequences

I want to acknowledge that many of the writers I work with are good hearted, compassionate, and caring individuals. They pursue the work they do because they truly want to help people and make the world a better place. However, like all of us, they live in a fat hating society and are influenced by anti-"obesity" rhetoric. When many fat individuals experience the "War on Obesity" as a war to eradicate them from existence, we must do better if we want to avoid harming the very people we want to help.

For those who are conducting research into weight and health, working to become health care professionals, or participating in continuing education credits, you can become better writers. Find good sources to guide your work and challenge them. Do not accept everything you read at face value. Select your words carefully and with compassion. Think about the experiences of fat individuals and, whenever possible, incorporate their own understanding of those experiences into your work. Do not assume you know how fat individuals experience the world. When you propose programs or policies, carefully consider how they might cause unforeseen and unintended harm.

Note

1 Note that sources referenced in examples are not included in the reference list for this chapter.

References

Alberts, B., Kirschner, M. W., Tilghman, S., & Varmus, H. (2014). Rescuing US biomedical research from its systemic flaws. *Proceedings of the National Academy of Sciences*, *111*(16), 5773–5777. https://doi.org/10.1073/pnas.1404402111

Anderson, M. S., Ronning, E. A., De Vries, R., & Martinson, B. C. (2007). The perverse effects of competition on scientists' work and relationships. *Science and Engineering Ethics*, *13*(4), 437–461. https://doi.org/10.1007/s11948-007-9042-5

Brown, H. (2012). *Fashioning a self from which to thrive: Negotiating size privilege as a fat woman learner at a small liberal arts college in the Midwest* [Doctoral dissertation]. Northern Illinois University, DeKalb, IL.

Brown, H. (2016). Fat studies in the field of higher education: Developing a theoretical framework and its implications for research and practice. In E. Carter & C. Russell (Eds.), *The fat pedagogy reader: Challenging weight-based oppression in education* (pp. 201–209). Peter Lang.

Brown, H. (2017). "There's always stomach on the table and then I gotta write!" Physical space and learning in fat college women. *Fat Studies: An Interdisciplinary Journal of Body Weight and Society, 7*(1), 11–20. https://doi.org/10.1080/21604851.2017.1360665

Casadevall, A., & Fang, F. (2012). Reforming science: Methodological and cultural reforms. *Infection and Immunity, 80*(3), 891–896. https://doi.org/10.1128/IAI.06183-11

Cooper, C. (1998). *Fat and proud: The politics of size.* The Women's Press.

Cooper, C. (2010). Fat studies: Mapping the field. *Sociology Compass, 4*(12), 1020–1034. https://doi.org/10.1111/j.1751-9020.2010.00336.x

Davis, M. S., Riske-Morris, M., & Diaz, S. R. (2007). Causal factors implicated in research misconduct: Evidence from ORI case files. *Science and Engineering Ethics, 13*(4), 395–414. https://doi.org/10.1007/s11948-007-9045-2

Dennett, C. (n.d.). The perils of person-first language. *Today's Dietitian.* https://www.todaysdietitian.com/enewsletter/enews_0118_01.shtml

Fanelli, D. (2009). How many scientists fabricate and falsify research? A systematic review and meta-analysis of survey data. *PLoS ONE, 4*(5), e5738. https://doi.org/10.1371/journal.pone.0005738

Fogel, R. B., Malhotra, A., Dalagiorgou, G., Robinson, M. K., Jakab, M., Kikinis, R., Pittman, S. D., & White, D. P. (2003). Anatomic and physiologic predictors of apnea severity in morbidly obese subjects. *Sleep, 26*(2), 150–155.

Garrett, C. K. (2017). Writing for the sciences: Lecture for the parallel computing summer research internship. *Los Alamos National Laboratory.* https://permalink.lanl.gov/object/tr?what=info:lanl-repo/lareport/LA-UR-17-25238

Gregg, A. (1957). *For future doctors.* University of Chicago Press.

Hamblin, J. (2018, September 24). A credibility crisis in food science: The fall of a prominent behavioral scientist tells of a system where research is judged not on merit, but on the attention it gets. *The Atlantic.* https://www.theatlantic.com/health/archive/2018/09/what-is-food-science/571105/

Harjunen, H. (2009). *Women and fat: Approaches to the social study of fatness.* (Unpublished doctoral dissertation.) University of Jyväskylä.

Harzing, A., & Kroonenberg, P. (2017). *The mystery of the phantom reference.* https://harzing.com/publications/white-papers/the-mystery-of-the-phantom-reference

Heath, H. III (2018). Writing for success. In J. Markovac, M. Kleinman, and M. Englesbe (Eds.), *Medical and scientific publishing: Author, editor, and reviewer perspectives* (pp. 93–101). https://doi.org/10.1016/B978-0-12-809969-8.00010-3

Journal of the American Medical Association. (1900). Medical literature and medical writing. *The Journal of the American Medical Association, XXXV*(10), 626–627. https://doi.org/10.1001/jama.1900.02460360032002

Kyle, T. K., & Puhl, R. M. (2014). Putting people first in obesity. *Obesity, 22*(5), 1211. https://doi.org/10.1002/oby.20727

Kobayashi, F. (2009). Academic achievement, BMI, and fast food intake of American and Japanese college students. *Nutrition and Food Science, 39*(5), 555–566. https://doi.org/10.1108/00346650910992213

Kotlikoff, M. I. (2018, September 20). *Statement of Cornell University Provost Michael I. Kotlikoff.* Cornel University. https://statements.cornell.edu/2018/20180920-statement-provost-michael-kotlikoff.cfm

Obesity Action Coalition (n.d.). *Weight bias: People-first language.* https://www.obesityaction.org/action-through-advocacy/weight-bias/people-first-language/

National Institutes of Health. (2020, February 24). Estimates of funding for various research, condition, and disease categories. https://report.nih.gov/categorical_spending.aspx

Palad, C. J., & Stanford, F. C. (2018). Use of people-first language with regard to obesity. *The American Journal of Clinical Nutrition, 108*(1), 201–203. https://doi.org/10.1093/ajcn/nqy076

Radovsky, S. S. (1979). Medical writing: Another look. *New England Journal of Medicine, 301*(3), 131–134. https://doi.org/10.1056/NEJM197907193010304

Savage, V., & Yeh, P. (2019, September 26). Novelist Cormac McCarthy's tips on how to write a great science paper. *Nature.* https://www.nature.com/articles/d41586-019-02918-5

Sargent, J. D., & Blanchflower, D. G. (1994). Obesity and stature in adolescence and earnings in young adulthood: Analysis of a British birth cohort. *Archives of Pediatrics & Adolescent Medicine, 148*(7), 681–687.

Singh, S., & McMahan, S. (2006). An evaluation of the relationship between academic performance and physical fitness measures in California schools. *Californian Journal of Health Promotion, 4*(2), 207–214.

Solovay, S., & Rothblum, E. (2009). Introduction. In E. Rothblum & S. Solovay (Eds.), *The fat studies reader* (pp. 1–7). New York University Press.

Spurlock, M. (Producer & Director). (2004). *Super size me* [Motion picture]. Samuel Goldwyn Films and Roadside Attractions.

Stephan, P. (2012). Perverse incentives. *Nature, 484*(7392), 29–31.

Teitelbaum, M. S. (2008). Research funding. Structural disequilibria in biomedical research. *Science, 321*(5889), 644–645.https://doi.org/10.1126/science.1160272

U.S. Department of Health and Human Services. (2009). Findings of scientific misconduct. *Federal Register, 74*(62), 14990–14991. https://www.govinfo.gov/content/pkg/FR-2009-04-02/pdf/E9-7406.pdf

Vastag, B. (2004). Obesity is now on everyone's plate. *JAMA, 291*(10), 1186–1188. https://doi.org/10.1001/jama.291.10.1186

Wann, M. (2009). Foreword: Fat studies: An invitation to revolution. In E. Rothblum & S. Solovay (Eds.), *The fat studies reader* (pp. ix–xxv). New York University Press.

11 Clinical revulsion

Combatting weight stigma by confronting provider disgust

Amanda K. Greene and Lisa M. Brownstone

Given that weight stigma does not originate in the fat body, but rather is built and reified in relational encounters between bodies, our intervention attends to the role of the health care provider's body in sustaining anti-fat bias during relational encounters with patients. Although providers may aspire to a disinterested clinical gaze, they are not immune to visceral aesthetic responses when engaging with fat individuals under their care. As "fat people are widely represented in popular culture and in interpersonal relationships as revolting" (Lebesco, 2004, p. 1) and anti-"obesity" public health campaigns frequently hinge on a "pedagogy of disgust" (Lupton, 2015, p. 2), these embodied interactions can become suffused with revulsion. Indeed, studies have shown that a significant percentage of providers—even health professionals who claim specialization in "obesity" and nutrition—are repulsed by their fat patients (Brown, 2006; Schwartz et al., 2003).

Revulsion is not benign. Providers' involuntary feelings of disgust are likely central to the enactment of weight stigma because, as Siebers argues in *Disability Aesthetics*, "aesthetic feelings of pleasure and disgust are difficult to separate from political feelings of acceptance and rejection" (2010, p. 60). There is also building evidence that disgust response is related to and even predictive of weight stigma and anti-fat bias, in addition to other stigma attitudes (e.g., Lieberman et al., 2012; Vartanian et al., 2016). Furthermore, momentary disgust has been shown experimentally to increase moral judgement (Pizarro et al., 2011; Schnall et al., 2008). As such, left unquestioned, provider disgust can play a role in the dismissal and judgement of fat patients' concerns. This, in turn, impacts access to care, care seeking, and quality of care for fat individuals (Phelan et al., 2015). Disgust, therefore, must be openly discussed, acknowledged, and dealt with among health care professionals, as it likely pervades health care settings and insidiously mutates into judgements, rejections, and biases. Health care provider training must help trainees and providers grapple directly and intentionally with their experiences of disgust, such that its negative impact on weight stigma and quality of care can be minimized.

Our chapter deepens this claim about the role of providers' feelings of revulsion in perpetuating anti-fat bias. We argue that because revulsion quickly slips into judgement and unrecognized biases, we must make space in training to (a) increase provider awareness of their own momentary disgust response, (b) build provider understanding of the negative impact that disgust has on clinical care

DOI: 10.4324/9781003057000-13

and stigma, and (c) create reflective spaces for providers to contend with and challenge their own disgust. Drawing on a rich body of interdisciplinary scholarship in Fat Studies, disability studies, aesthetic theory, moral psychology, and public health, as well as Dr. Brownstone's clinical work on dismantling internalized weight stigma among patients and staff in eating disorder treatment settings, we propose that future health care provider training intervene at the level of disgust in order to minimize enactment of weight stigma in health care.

Theories of disgust

Before turning to clinical revulsion specifically, it is worth sitting a little longer with the often-uncomfortable notion of disgust itself. Disgust may seem like a fairly benign affect in comparison to feelings like anger and fear that are more often associated with inducing harm. Expressions of disgust are common in everyday conversations, rhetorical tools deployed to move past something without looking too closely (e.g., "that sexist behavior disgusts me."). As a result, the violence spurred by disgust responses might at first appear to be nothing more than a glancing blow.

Nevertheless, the theoretical history of disgust reveals a different story in which disgust is not about mere avoidance but instead visceral rejection. Our review of the literature in this section details with why disgust is critically important to understanding clinical encounters and is especially relevant when it comes to the fat body. While a comprehensive overview of the rich body of scholarship on disgust is clearly outside of the scope of this chapter, we offer a basic framework for our intervention by quickly synthesizing three different theoretical orientations toward disgust that we term pathogenic, moral, and aesthetic.

Pathogenic instinct

Many conceptions of disgust hinge on its evolutionary utility as a protective force. A notion of "core disgust" has developed based on the idea that certain forms of disgust are ingrained, embodied responses that transcend cultural specificity (Rozin et al., 1999). Curtis et al. (2011) succinctly summarize this position as follows:

> Disgust is an evolved psychological system for protecting organisms from infection through disease avoidant behaviour. This 'behavioural immune system,' present in a diverse array of species, exhibits universal features that orchestrate hygienic behaviour in response to cues of risk of contact with pathogens. (p. 2)

Disgust's visceral impact trains humans to regularly avoid substances and objects that are associated with contamination by harmful pathogens and parasites (Chapman & Anderson, 2012). Given this self-protective impulse, Haidt et al. evocatively label core disgust the "guardian to the temple of the body" (1994, p. 114). The intensity of disgust as a boundary-creating, self-preserving impulse helps link it to notions of health and illness beyond particular pathological substances (Haidt et al., 1994).

It is also worth noting that instinctual pathogenic disgust is particularly connected to oral rejection given how oral consumption is a primary and incredibly intimate way in which "materials outside of the self are taken into the self" (Rozin et al., 1999, p. 432). Some researchers also argue that disgust is so directly linked to orality because it originated first in the related idea of "distaste—a mechanism that served to warn against the consumption of potentially toxic substances (Chapman et al., 2009, 2017). This link is, of course, clearly evident in the term's English etymology. Thus, the policing of oral consumption lies at the core of the prophylactic bodily knowledge associated with disgust.

Moral feeling

Disgust's reification of the boundaries between self and dangerous environments is a major reason why disgust is so easily recruited into moral judgements. This value-driven aspect of disgust has been explored in a large body of empirical moral psychology research. Hutcherson and Gross (2011), for example, label disgust a "moral emotion." In their account, moral disgust parallels core disgust as a mechanism for boundary setting and self-protection; the main function of moral disgust is to "mark individuals whose behavior suggests that they represent a threat and avoid them, thereby reducing the risk of exposure to harm" (Hutcherson & Gross, 2011, p. 720). This basic protective instinct does not always accurately reflect the reality of "threatening" situations. Moral psychology literature shows that elicitation of disgust seems to increase the severity of moral judgements even when the scenarios being judged do not involve harm (e.g., Wheatley & Haidt, 2005).

Haidt et al. (1997) elaborated on the way core disgust extends into broader sociocultural spheres by arguing that disgust is a form of embodied cognition. As an embodied rejection system, disgust can be harnessed into rejections beyond its initial evolutionary response to pathogens. In other words, "human societies take advantage of the schemata of core disgust in constructing their moral and social lives, and in socializing their children about what to avoid" (Haidt et al., 1997, p. 124). This ready-made, strongly-felt schema lends itself as a way of demarcating us versus them and deciding who or what is labeled "Other" within a given sociocultural context (Seidman, 2013). Further supporting these claims that "core disgust" and "moral disgust" are really driven by the same brand of embodied cognition, empirical research has shown that feelings of disgust can measurably amplify the intensity of moral judgements. (Pizarro et al., 2011; Schnall et al., 2008)

Aesthetic unreadability

An aesthetic account of disgust frequently intersects with moral accounts that frame disgust as an embodied technology of judgement. Kant's famous aesthetic treatise is after all, titled *The Critique of Judgement*. Within a Kantian paradigm the disgusting "disposes us and compels us to decisively repel that which runs counter to morality, is unfree, and appears in disharmony with the 'wholesome' and 'beautiful' coherence of nature" (Kant, 1790, as cited in Menninghaus, 2003,

p. 116). Or, as disability studies scholar, Siebers (2010), more directly frames it, "aesthetic feelings of pleasure and disgust are difficult to separate from political feelings of acceptance and rejection" (p. 60).

However, despite this overlap between aesthetics and morality, turning to relational encounters and aesthetic responses to the physical body adds a richer, more intimate and individual dimension than sweeping cultural diagnoses. This is particularly true when we approach aesthetics as a phenomenon that "tracks the sensations that some bodies feel in the presence of other bodies" (Siebers, 2010, p. 1) as opposed to a disinterested mode of artistic judgement. This thinking also has a direct bearing on clinical encounters because aesthetically disgust can only be disgusting and evades "readership." By implication, it can obstruct the clinician's ability to read the body of their patient to the level that care and diagnosis require.

Kant names three categories of objects that elicit an aesthetic response from the viewer. While the beautiful and the sublime are the most heavily conceptualized, the disgusting is isolated as having its own unique set of aesthetic effects. The disgusting is not just "not beautiful," he argues "there is only one kind of ugliness that cannot be presented in conformity with nature without obliterating all aesthetic liking and hence artistic beauty" (Kant, 1790, as cited in Menninghaus, 2003, p. 9). In other words, disgust makes representation impossible on some level. Disgust prevents the disgusting object from being seen in any light or with any characteristics of pleasure or liking and, as a result, cannot be recognized by the viewer except as disgusting. With its characteristic gesture of "looking away" disgust forecloses prolonged engagement or connection before it begins.

Existing alongside and in tension with this distancing, aesthetic disgust is also often defined by unwanted contact and contagion as opposed to a fully achieved avoidance. For Nietzsche, for example, the experience of encountering a disgusting object always ends up turning into disgust at the self and internalized shame at one's own animality and corporeality (Nietzsche, 1887, as cited in Menninghaus, 2003, p. 156). Disgust in this light is so powerful because it is an impulse to reject something that is not simply entirely, neatly "other" but has also already been internalized as a pathological part of the self. Or, to look at this seemingly contagious aesthetic encounter in different terms, Ahmed (2013) describes disgust as characterized by "stickiness." Disgust is a violent reaction against something that threatens to stick to (or has already left its sticky residue on) the observer. As a result, an attempt to extricate oneself can easily turn into an assault against one's own body. Counterintuitively, in the attempt to reinforce its boundaries, the body is itself convulsed and affected with disgust.

Disgust and fat

Pop culture

These core ontological characteristics of disgust are, of course, not inherently connected to the fat body in spite of the fact that some scholars have unfortunately tried to rationalize this response as natural. However, the prevalence of cultural messaging that associates fat bodies with disgust frequently normalizes this connection in contemporary western society. As LeBesco (2004) asserts "fat people are widely represented in popular culture and interpersonal interactions as revolting—they are agents of abhorrence and disgust" (LeBesco, 2004, p. 1.) Fat Studies scholars have compellingly drawn attention to the wide range of ways in which the fat body is negatively stigmatized and pathologized in the media through content analyses of news, television, and YouTube videos (Boero, 2007; Campos et al., 2006; Himes & Thompson, 2007; Yoo & Kim, 2012).

More than just nebulous negative stereotypes about the health and character of fat people, though, a number of other studies have illuminated the ways in which disgust is explicitly deployed in popular media that depicts fat bodies. Drawing on recent affect theory in tandem with the idea of biopolitics, Rich (2011) argues that weight-loss focused reality television shows are a political technology that makes fat bodies into "bad bodies." In the dialogue she quotes to support this claim, disgust is a recurring theme and is even frequently directly named. Inthorn and Boyce's (2010) analysis of anti-"obesity" messaging on British television emphasizes how the medical experts who appear in this content often openly display disgust at the fat body. They emphasize that "on tv the 'obese' body becomes an object of ridicule and disgust instead of simply a public health problem" (p. 84). While disgust is often explicitly performed or named in these contexts, plenty of other tropes that stick to depictions of fat bodies in popular culture like contagion, "war against obesity," and toxic fat all reinforce the fat body as something that must be kept at a distance that poses a pathological threat. Similarly, Jillian Michaels, the self-proclaimed nutritionist and former fitness coach on *The Biggest Loser* proclaimed that "it goes too far to glamorize 'obesity' ... I don't celebrate anyone being 'overweight,' because it's unhealthy" when critiquing Lizzo's positive stance regarding her own larger body (KTLA 5, 2020). As such, Michaels proclaims that larger bodies are not worthy of celebration, as they are to be feared as potential disease markers.

The connection between disgust and the fat body is also explicitly taught and supported by official medical messaging. Lupton's (2015) influential coinage of the "pedagogy of disgust" shows how frequently disgust is deliberately deployed in public health campaigns. The "war on obesity" is her prime example, clearly articulating how the fat body is authoritatively labeled disgusting and offensive. Furthermore, Leahy (2012) writes that disgust is "actively mobilized in health education classroom spaces" as part of pedagogies meant to address the "obesity" epidemic (p.179). For example, Atlanta's anti-childhood "obesity" campaign "Strong4Life" employs images of children in larger bodies with quotes such as "Fat Kids Become Fat Adults" and "It's hard to be a little girl if you're not" (Teegardin, 2012). These messages clearly disconnect children from their youth and represent them as feared medical outcomes that are quickly becoming adult burdens on society. We can see in this campaign the elicitation of pathogen and moral disgust.

Weight stigma

O'Brian et al. (2016) claim that, given how disgust sensitivity and "obesity" stigma are linked, disgust is a prominent candidate for understanding anti-fat bias. Evidence suggests that weight stigma elicits both pathogenic and moral disgust (Lieberman et al., 2012). Furthermore, those with higher pathogen disgust sensitivity have more pronounced anti-fat bias, particularly after viewing images of "obese" individuals (Park et al., 2007). Notably, disgust has also been found to be a mediator in the relationship between the body size of a person being viewed and the participant's weight stigma experience (Vartanian et al., 2016). Looking more closely at mechanisms of disgust, Vartanian (2010) found that weight stigma is even further connected to disgust experience when individuals perceive "obesity" as being within a person's behavioral control. This may relate to moral disgust, as theories of moral disgust posit that disgust functions to help us determine who has more intrinsic moral value and thus can be viewed as safe for engagement. Additionally, given "obesity" epidemic rhetoric, fat bodies have been framed as equivalent to disease. As such, people's bodies are deemed disease states and locations for public health crisis interventions. It is not surprising that such bodies elicit varying types of disgust response among the general population given the links between pathogen fear, morality and disgust as described throughout this chapter.

Clinical responses

Pertinent to the current chapter, however, it is not just the general public that experiences disgust response when faced with reminders of weight stigma attitudes (e.g., seeing fat bodies). Health care providers have also been shown to experience a similar disgust response to their patients in larger bodies (Brown, 2006). Studies also show more broadly that providers are less likely to experience "respect," "hope," and "competence" to treat their larger bodied patients (e.g., Beames et al., 2016; Puhl, Latner et al., 2014; Schwartz et al., 2003). And this pattern does not appear to be changing in younger trainees, as health care professional trainees observe weight bias regularly among peers, health care providers and instructors, and experience their own "pessimism" and "frustration" regarding the treatment of higher weight individuals (Puhl, Luedicke, et al., 2014). Similarly, the majority of large sample of medical students from a variety of medical schools were found to hold implicit (74%) and explicit (67%) weight stigma attitudes (Phelan et al., 2015). These statistics are concerning given the existing literature on stigma attitudes among providers predicting worse treatment outcomes and patient care (Penner et al., 2018). Clearly, rising health care providers need education on competent care for patients with all body sizes and shapes.

While preliminary efforts have been made to build interventions aimed at decreasing weight stigma among trainees and providers, and have shown preliminary promise (Poustchi et al., 2013; Wiese et al., 1992), work in this area is very much in its early stages. There have been efforts, however, to decrease weight stigma among the general population and college samples. Some of these interventions have focused on changing beliefs about the controllability of weight by means of education about genetic or psychological correlates of higher weight status (Anesbury & Tiggeman, 2000; Khan et al., 2018). Others have worked to reduce weight stigma by means of empathy building and perspective taking practice (Gapinski et al., 2006; Gloor & Puhl, 2016). A different set of studies looked at social consensus as a place for intervention to challenge weight stigma beliefs (e.g., by telling participants that their anti-fat belief is higher than that of most others, which in turn led to decreased reporting of weight stigma; Puhl et al., 2005; Zitek & Hebl, 2007). Another study found that eliciting cognitive dissonance among participants led to decreased weight bias (Ciao & Latner, 2011). As such, multiple targets of intervention have been identified that seem to have an impact on momentary reporting of weight stigma. How can we build upon such findings and further develop interventions specifically aimed for individuals providing health care to individuals of all sizes and size histories?

Interventions in clinical revulsion

Intellectual and cognitive anti-weight stigma interventions (e.g., belief challenging, empathy building, and social consensus and cognitive dissonance manipulation) may help providers dismantle weight stigma, particularly as it affects care of patients. However, given the existing literature, it is clear that weight stigma emerges from a less conscious source linked to evolutionary, relational, survival, and aesthetic roots (i.e., one pathway by which this happens is the experience of disgust). We must address these deeper roots with health care provider trainees as part of disrupting the suboptimal care that larger bodied individuals are getting in our existing medical system.

Interventions meant to mitigate providers' weight stigma must incorporate intellectual and affective engagement for maximal effect. We must help providers in training recognize and own their affective responses even if such responses are shameful to admit (e.g., clinical revulsion). We can draw upon existing multicultural training frameworks that prompt individuals to build reflective capacity to witness their own resistance to learning about parts of self that perhaps exist in contrast to conscious personal values. Providers should be taught to label and acknowledge their own level of privilege related to body size, including realizing their comparative access to spaces, power, compassion, and respect in our existing world due to the size of their body. To gain this sort of self-reflective capacity, providers may need to build internal dissonance and willingness to be uncomfortable with reflexive responses that run counter to core values (e.g., values that prompted them to pursue a career in health care, such as care, service, justice). We could help provider trainees begin to recognize and challenge their disgust responses by providing an intellectual frame for why they may have this automatic response given the fat phobic diet culture in which they have been socialized. Such an approach would be in keeping with Kinavey and Cool's (2019) "body liberation" framework which they propose psychotherapists should promote as mental health providers. Perhaps health care providers from all disciplines could be educated in anti-diet culture frameworks that bring about cognitive dissonance regarding habitual disgust response to bodies that may represent a deviance from diet culture.

New disgust pedagogies

Dr. Brownstone developed curriculum at a Partial Hospitalization Program/Intensive Outpatient eating disorder program aimed at helping patients with either current or history of weight stigma experience to help them process and dismantle their internalized experience of weight stigma (for more details about this curriculum see Brownstone et al., 2021). Patients learned about the power of challenging existing language paradigms (e.g., using small, large, and size-privilege labels in lieu of "obese," "overweight," and other words that conjure disease models of the body) to describe bodies of varied and diverse shapes and sizes (as described by Evans (2018)). Patients also worked on engaging in experiences that they may have avoided prior to such a group setting (e.g., ordering an "unhealthy" snack at a stereotypically "healthy" store like Whole Foods, trying on clothing in the correct size at a local thrift store despite shame). Such experiences allowed patients to find common ground related to ways that weight stigma has gotten in the way of a fully lived life. Patients reported increasing empowerment to notice and de-value their own thoughts/beliefs that they began to recognize are products of anti-fat oppression. They did so by allowing themselves to learn new ways of understanding the definition of "health" and "beauty" to encompass more than equivalence to body size/shape.

It is likely that provider trainees would benefit from similar joining experiences related to their own less than pride-inducing experiences with patients who are in larger bodies, not to mention how weight stigma and diet culture fuel their own self-disgust regarding bodies. This sort of intervention would perhaps help disrupt the less conscious and automatic processes that emerge in the patient encounter. For example, provider trainees could be given the opportunity to have both private and small group reflective spaces to notice their own disgust responses, slow them down, and write about where such responses may "come from." Given the educational settings that may not include safe processing spaces for the most personal of disclosures, some of these reflections could be private (stated so in the introduction to the reflective exercise), while others could be presented as opportunities to reveal more personally with the larger group. For example, trainees could answer the prompt: "many individuals experience automatic disgust or revulsion when looking at humans in larger bodies. Why do you think individuals experience this disgust? If you were to feel disgust, where might it stem from in your own history?" These questions hold varying levels of opportunity to engage anywhere from intellectually to emotionally. Trainees would benefit from such options that allow for self- selection regarding how personal they get in their self-disclosures.

Conclusion(s)

In the current chapter, we propose one potential point of intervention that could help bring providers closer to battling their own implicit weight stigma attitudes that permeate their patient care. Although disgust at fat bodies is learned in particular sociocultural contexts as opposed to being innate, disgust is nevertheless a powerfully visceral, disruptive feeling that can overwhelm intellectual judgement and undermine the ideal of a neutral, disinterested gaze. By implication, we must consider how to intervene at the level of automatic disgust, which could in turn disrupt such a process at a deeper level than one that merely addresses the information/intellectual components of weight stigma. Such interventions should increase provider awareness of their own momentary disgust response, build understanding of how disgust creates stigma, and create reflective spaces for providers to contend with and challenge their own disgust.

Disgust is not benign. The stakes are high when clinicians reflexively turn away from fat bodies, when these bodies are unconsciously approached as infectious, immoral, or illegible. While there is no "easy fix" to simply eliminate clinical revulsion given how profoundly disgust and fatness have been entangled within popular culture and medical rhetoric, it is imperative to confront this intense affect because of how it materially reverberates into provider-patient interactions and into substandard care. Only by supporting the difficult, uncomfortable work of facing and feeling disgust can we begin to mitigate its insidious negative health impacts and open new pathways toward more just and effective futures of care.

References

Ahmed, S. (2013). *The cultural politics of emotion*. Routledge.

Anesbury, T., & Tiggemann, M. (2000). An attempt to reduce negative stereotyping of obesity in children by changing controllability beliefs. *Health Education Research, 15*(2), 145–152.

Beames, J. R., Black, J. J., & Vartanian, L. R. (2016). Prejudice toward individuals with obesity: Evidence for a pro-effort bias. *Journal of Experimental Psychology: Applied, 22*(2), 184.

Boero, N. (2007). All the news that's fat to print: The American "obesity epidemic" and the media. *Qualitative Sociology, 30*(1), 41–60. https://doi.org/10.1007/s11133-006-9010-4

Brown, I. (2006). Nurses' attitudes towards adult patients who are obese: Literature review. *Journal of Advanced Nursing, 53*(2), 221–232. https://doi.org/10.1111/j.1365-2648.2006.03718.x

Brownstone, L. M., Kelly, D. A., Ko, S. J., Jasper, M. L., Sumlin, L., Hall, J., Anderson, E., & Goffredi, A. (2021, March 17). Dismantling weight stigma: A group intervention in a partial hospitalization and intensive outpatient eating disorder treatment program. *Psychotherapy*. https://doi.org/10.1037/pst0000358

Campos, P., Saguy, A., Ernsberger, P., Oliver, E., & Gaesser, G. (2006). The epidemiology of overweight and obesity: Public health crisis or moral panic? *International Journal of Epidemiology, 35*(1), 55–60. https://doi.org/10.1093/ije/dyi254

Chapman, H. A., & Anderson, A. K. (2012). Understanding disgust. *Annals of the New York Academy of Sciences, 1251*(1), 62–76. https://doi.org/10.1111/j.1749-6632.2011.06369.x

Chapman, H. A., Kim, D. A., Susskind, J. M., & Anderson, A. K. (2009). In bad taste: Evidence for the oral origins of moral disgust. *Science*, 323(5918), 1222–1226. https://doi.org/10.1126/science.1165565

Chapman, H. A., Lee, D. H., Susskind, J. M., Bartlett, M. S., & Anderson, A. K. (2017). The face of distaste: A preliminary study. *Chemical Senses*, 42(6), 457–463. https://doi.org/10.1093/chemse/bjx024

Ciao, A. C., & Latner, J. D. (2011). Reducing obesity stigma: The effectiveness of cognitive dissonance and social consensus interventions. *Obesity*, 19(9), 1768–1774.

Curtis, V., De Barra, M., & Aunger, R. (2011). Disgust as an adaptive system for disease avoidance behaviour. *Philosophical Transactions of the Royal Society B: Biological Sciences*, 366(1563), 389–401. https://doi.org/10.1098/rstb.2010.0117

Evans, M. (2018, February 18). *Dismantling weight stigma one word at a time*. Marci RD Blog. https://marcird.com/dismantling-stigma-one-word-at-a-time/

Gapinski, K. D., Schwartz, M. B., & Brownell, K. D. (2006). Can television change anti-fat attitudes and behavior? *Journal of Applied Biobehavioral Research*, 11(1), 1–28.

Gloor, J. L., & Puhl, R. M. (2016). Empathy and perspective-taking: Examination and comparison of strategies to reduce weight stigma. *Stigma and Health*, 1(4), 269.

Haidt, J., McCauley, C., & Rozin, P. (1994). Individual differences in sensitivity to disgust: A scale sampling seven domains of disgust elicitors. *Personality and Individual Differences*, 16(5), 701–713. https://doi.org/10.1016/0191-8869(94)90212-7

Haidt, J., Rozin, P., McCauley, C., & Imada, S. (1997). Body, psyche, and culture: The relationship between disgust and morality. *Psychology and Developing Societies*, 9(1), 107–131.

Himes, S. M., & Thompson, J. K. (2007). Fat stigmatization in television shows and movies: A content analysis. *Obesity*, 15(3), 712–718. https://doi.org/10.1038/oby.2007.635

Hutcherson, C. A., & Gross, J. J. (2011). The moral emotions: A social-functionalist account of anger, disgust, and contempt. *Journal of Personality and Social Psychology*, 100(4), 719.

Inthorn, S., & Boyce, T. (2010). 'It's disgusting how much salt you eat!' Television discourses of obesity, health and morality. *International Journal of Cultural Studies*, 13(1), 83–100. https://doi.org/10.1177%2F1367877909348540

Khan, S. S., Tarrant, M., Weston, D., Shah, P., & Farrow, C. (2018). Can raising awareness about the psychological causes of obesity reduce obesity stigma? *Health Communication*, 33(5), 585–592.

Kinavey, H., & Cool, C. (2019). The broken lens: How anti-fat bias in psychotherapy is harming our clients and what to do about it. *Women & Therapy*, 42(1–2), 116–130.

KTLA 5. (2020, January 15). *"It's Science." Exasperated Jillian Michaels explains her comments about diets, weight & Lizzo*. [Video File.] https://youtu.be/_IqhqwuLGpE

Leahy, D. (2012). Disgusting pedagogies. In J. Wright & V. Harwood (Eds.), *Biopolitics and the 'obesity epidemic': Governing bodies* (pp. 180–190). Routledge.

LeBesco, K. (2004). *Revolting bodies? The struggle to redefine fat identity*. University of Massachusetts Press.

Lieberman, D. L., Tybur, J. M., & Latner, J. D. (2012). Disgust sensitivity, obesity stigma, and gender: Contamination psychology predicts weight bias for women, not men. *Obesity*, 20(9), 1803–1814. https://doi.org/10.1038/oby.2011.247

Lupton, D. (2015). The pedagogy of disgust: The ethical, moral and political implications of using disgust in public health campaigns. *Critical Public Health*, 25(1), 4–14. https://doi.org/10.1080/09581596.2014.885115

Menninghaus, W. (2003). *Disgust: Theory and history of a strong sensation*. SUNY Press.

O'Brien, K. S., Latner, J. D., Puhl, R. M., Vartanian, L. R., Giles, C., Griva, K., & Carter, A. (2016). The relationship between weight stigma and eating behavior is explained by weight bias internalization and psychological distress. *Appetite, 102*, 70–76.

Park, J. H., Schaller, M., & Crandall, C. S. (2007). Pathogen-avoidance mechanisms and the stigmatization of obese people. *Evolution and Human Behavior, 28*(6), 410–414. https://doi.org/10.1016/j.evolhumbehav.2007.05.008

Penner, L. A., Phelan, S. M., Earnshaw, V., Albrecht, T. L., & Dovidio, J. F. (2018). Patient stigma, medical interactions, and health care disparities: A selective review, In B. Major, J. F. Dovidio, & B. G. Link (Eds.), *The Oxford handbook of stigma, discrimination, and health* (pp. 183–202). Oxford University Press.

Phelan, S. M., Burgess, D. J., Yeazel, M. W., Hellerstedt, W. L., Griffin, J. M., & van Ryn, M. (2015). Impact of weight bias and stigma on quality of care and outcomes for patients with obesity. *Obesity Reviews, 16*(4), 319–326.

Pizarro, D., Inbar, Y., & Helion, C. (2011). On disgust and moral judgment. *Emotion Review, 3*(3), 267–268.

Poustchi, Y., Saks, N. S., Piasecki, A. K., Hahn, K. A., & Ferrante, J. M. (2013). Brief intervention effective in reducing weight bias in medical students. *Family Medicine, 45*(5), 345.

Puhl, R. M., Latner, J. D., King, K. M., & Luedicke, J. (2014). Weight bias among professionals treating eating disorders: Attitudes about treatment and perceived patient outcomes. *International Journal of Eating Disorders, 47*(1), 65–75. https://doi.org/10.1002/eat.22186

Puhl, R. M., Schwartz, M. B., & Brownell, K. D. (2005). Impact of perceived consensus on stereotypes about obese people: A new approach for reducing bias. *Health Psychology, 24*(5), 517.

Rich, E. (2011). "I see her being obesed!": Public pedagogy, reality media and the obesity crisis. *Health, 15*(1), 3–21. https://doi.org/10.1177%2F1363459309358127

Rozin, P., Haidt, J., & McCauley, C. R. (1999). Disgust: The body and soul emotion. In T. Dalgleish & M. Power (Eds.), *Handbook of cognition and emotion* (pp. 429–445). John Wiley & Sons.

Schnall, S., Haidt, J., Clore, G. L., & Jordan, A. H. (2008). Disgust as embodied moral judgment. *Personality and Social Psychology Bulletin, 34*(8), 1096–1109.

Schwartz, M. B., Chambliss, H. O. N., Brownell, K. D., Blair, S. N., & Billington, C. (2003). Weight bias among health professionals specializing in obesity. *Obesity Research, 11*(9), 1033–1039. https://doi.org/10.1038/oby.2003.142

Seidman, S. (2013) Defilement and disgust: Theorizing the other. *American Journal of Cultural Sociology, 1*, 3–25. https://doi.org/10.1057/ajcs.2012.3

Siebers, T. (2010). *Disability aesthetics*. University of Michigan Press.

Teegardin, C. (2012, January 3). *Grim childhood obesity ads stir critics*. College of Public Health, University of Georgia. https://publichealth.uga.edu/grim-childhood-obesity-ads-stir-critics/#:~:text=Grim%20childhood%20obesity%20ads%20stir%20critics.%20Children%E2%80%99s%20Healthcare,families%20to%20recognize%20the%20widespread%20public%20health%20problem

Vartanian, L. R. (2010). Disgust and perceived control in attitudes toward obese people. *International Journal of Obesity, 34*(8), 1302–1307. https://doi.org/10.1038/ijo.2010.45

Vartanian, L. R., Trewartha, T., & Vanman, E. J. (2016). Disgust predicts prejudice and discrimination toward individuals with obesity. *Journal of Applied Social Psychology, 46*(6), 369–375. https://doi.org/10.1111/jasp.12370

Wheatley, T., & Haidt, J. (2005). Hypnotic disgust makes moral judgments more severe. *Psychological Science*, *16*(10), 780–784. https://doi.org/10.1111%2Fj.1467-9280.2005.01614.x

Wiese, H. J., Wilson, J. F., Jones, R. A., & Neises, M. (1992). Obesity stigma reduction in medical students. *International Journal of Obesity and Related Metabolic Disorders: Journal of the International Association for the Study of Obesity*, *16*(11), 859–868.

Yoo, J. H., & Kim, J. (2012). Obesity in the new media: A content analysis of obesity videos on YouTube. *Health Communication*, *27*(1), 86–97. https://doi.org/10.1080/10410236.2011.569003

Zitek, E. M., & Hebl, M. R. (2007). The role of social norm clarity in the influenced expression of prejudice over time. *Journal of Experimental Social Psychology*, *43*(6), 867–876.

12 Anti-fat bias in evidence-based psychotherapies for eating disorders

Can they be adapted to address the harm?

Rachel Millner and Lauren Muhlheim

Evidence-based psychotherapies such as family-based treatment (FBT), cognitive behavioral therapy (CBT), and dialectical behavioral therapy (DBT) are often viewed as the treatment methods of choice for individuals with eating disorders. However, they have been primarily studied among patients in smaller bodies and as they are commonly delivered, these treatment methods reinforce weight stigma. Many of the components of these evidence-based psychotherapies perpetuate anti-fat bias and are harmful to fat people. These treatment models are then taught to new clinicians entering the field, perpetuating the cycle of harm. When the treatments most often recommended for people with eating disorders are in fact harmful to a large portion of that group, we must look at the treatments themselves and decide if they can be changed to be weight inclusive—or if we need to abandon them altogether.

Evidence-based treatments overview

Most of the research studies on psychotherapy for eating disorders have focused on one of two groups. One set of studies has focused on traditional low to "normal" body mass index (BMI) weight patient groups with anorexia or bulimia. These studies have generally excluded patients in higher weight bodies because diagnostic criteria until 2013 required a low body weight for diagnosis of anorexia nervosa, and because fat bias led to the assumption that people in higher weight bodies could only experience binge eating disorder. The second set of studies has focused on people in higher weight bodies; these have often presumed binge eating disorder and included a focus on stopping bingeing, followed by a module on behavioral weight loss.

CBT (Fairburn et al., 1993) has been the psychological treatment most studied and validated for adults with eating disorders (including bulimia nervosa, binge eating disorder, and other specified feeding or eating disorders). It also has support for the treatment of adults with anorexia nervosa. FBT is the psychological treatment with the most support for treatment of adolescents with anorexia nervosa and also has support for adolescents with bulimia nervosa. Although less studied, there is also support for DBT for the treatment of eating disorders.

DOI: 10.4324/9781003057000-14

Since as far back as the 1950s, we have known that diets don't work. Stunkard (1958) stated that among people who are pursuing weight loss, "most will not lose weight and of those who do lose weight, most will regain it" (p. 79). A more recent comprehensive analysis on weight-loss diets (Mann et al., 2007) found that one-third to two-thirds of dieters re-gain more weight than they lost; it further noted that this was likely an underestimation due to research methodological flaws that biased the studies in the direction of showing weight loss. Diet culture's focus on weight loss at any cost has not turned fat people into thin people, but it has contributed to food preoccupation, body preoccupation, and weight cycling. Diets are often promoted as a way for people to improve "health," but evidence indicates that diet-driven weight change, if any, does not result in improved health (Mann et al., 2007). Furthermore, weight cycling (gaining and losing weight repeatedly) can contribute to medical problems such as insulin resistance, hypertension, and inflammation (Bacon & Aphramor, 2011).

Diets are associated with an increased risk of developing an eating disorder and the younger a person starts dieting, the higher the risk of developing an eating disorder (Neumark-Sztainer et al., 2011). When higher-weight people lose weight, they are often congratulated and praised. Many higher-weight people who appear to "successfully" lose weight are engaging in eating behaviors that would be considered disordered in someone of a lower weight. As Neumark-Sztainer (2015) noted in her editorial in the *Journal of Adolescent Health*:

> individuals who live in larger bodies but have serious restrictive eating disorders may not be taken as seriously as needs to happen by family members and by the health care system, may face issues such as disbelief by others that they are 'really consuming so few calories,' may not be adequately covered in terms of insurance for treatment, and may not be getting the treatment that they so desperately need. (p. 2)

Weight bias and stigma are present in every part of our culture. Health care settings and the eating disorder field are no exceptions. Weight bias among health care providers is well documented (Brownell et al., 2005). One of the only studies looking specifically at weight bias among eating disorder providers found that weight bias among these providers exists at a rate similar to other health care providers (Puhl et al., 2014). Eating disorder providers who endorsed a high level of weight bias not only had negative attitudes toward patients in higher-weight bodies, but they also reported poorer treatment outcomes compared to providers who reported less weight bias. In addition, this study showed a significantly higher attrition rate than other weight-bias studies conducted by the authors, and the attrition rate among eating disorder providers was highest when they were asked about their own attitudes toward patients in larger bodies.

Health at Every Size (HAES™) is offered as an alternative to the weight-centric model of health care. HAES is a weight inclusive model that takes the focus off of weight and directly opposes recommendations for weight loss. HAES recognizes the ways in which access, marginalization and oppression impact health outcomes and uses a social justice framework to understand "health" and health outcomes. HAES providers decouple health and weight while valuing body autonomy and choice in care (Burgard, 2009).

Current evidence-based treatment is not grounded in HAES and many of the recommendations in their treatment models are inherently weight stigmatizing. Common recommendations, including food journaling, calculating BMI, and weight exposures, fail to address the trauma many higher weight people have experienced due to weight stigma and can contribute to eating disordered behaviors. If evidence-based treatment is going to be offered as a treatment modality, changes must be made to remove weight bias from the models, or they will perpetuate harm for clients, particularly those in higher weight bodies. Evidence-based practice in mental health rests on three pillars: best available research; clinical expertise; and patient characteristics, culture, and preferences. Morales and Norcross (2010) offer a framework for applying evidence-based treatments to populations not included in the clinical trials for the treatments. Although they don't specifically address size diversity in the paper, we can extend their discussion.

Morales and Norcross (2010) framed the problem as follows: "In working with racial and ethnic minority patients, psychotherapists frequently confront a clinical dilemma. Should I use a research-supported treatment even if it has not been validated on patients of the same race or ethnicity as my patient?" (pp. 825–826). They conclude that practitioners have essentially three options for any particular patient with regard to a research-supported treatment: adopt it, adapt it, or abandon it. They recommend we *adopt* it when we believe the fit is good enough for this particular patient in this context. We *adapt* it when we believe it has utility, but does not seem adequate for this particular patient, problem, or situation. Finally, we might *abandon* it when we believe it does not apply to the particular patient or might not produce the desired results.

All evidence-based treatments for eating disorders were developed for thin or "normal weight," primarily affluent White cisgender females—and then they were applied to everyone else. Weight-loss regimens were not a part of these treatments, and were only added when the treatments were adapted to larger patients. Might the treatments be weight-biased as they are manualized or practiced? Might they be harming patients in larger bodies—or patients in any size body?

Analysis of specific treatment models

CBT

In its purely theoretical form, CBT focuses on helping individuals understand the connections and interactions among their thoughts, feelings, and behavior. This is entirely weight neutral in theory yet, in the application of this theory to eating disorders, weight stigma has entered the framework.

Some of the key elements in CBT for eating disorders include psychoeducation; establishing regular eating and self-monitoring; interrupting eating disorder behaviors (dieting, binge eating, and compensatory behaviors); developing alternative coping skills; addressing the over-evaluation of shape and weight; confronting dietary rules; and addressing perfectionism, low self-esteem, and interpersonal problems. Weekly weighing is also a core component.

In reviewing CBT manuals and workbooks, we found a significant weight bias. For example, there are CBT therapies specifically for weight loss. *Cognitive Behavioral Treatment of Obesity: A Clinician's Guide* by Cooper et al. (2003) is one example. Fairburn (2008) defined "obesity" as a medical disorder and suggested choosing between treating the eating disorder or addressing weight via his other book "and this might, or might not, simultaneously result in cessation of the binge eating" (p. 253).

Even as Fairburn recognizes that weight loss is inadvisable for people with bulimia, he inexplicably encourages it in patients with binge eating. "Weight loss treatments are inadvisable with patients with bulimia nervosa, however, as they intensify dietary restraint, one of the major causes of their binge-eating" (Fairburn, 2008, p. 253). But for patients who are "obese," "the other option is to treat the eating disorder first, the goal being to give patients control over their eating, and then they can consider tackling their weight" (Fairburn, 2008, p. 253).

In manuals and workbooks for eating disorders, we noticed a number of fat-phobic themes. For instance, many recognize that dietary restraint is a key problem in bulimia nervosa—stating that weight loss treatment is "inadvisable" for bulimia—but fail to recognize its role in maintaining binge eating disorder. The difference between the two disorders is that binge eating disorder is more commonly assumed to afflict people in larger bodies.

These texts often fail to recognize natural diversity of body weights and pathologize people in larger bodies. Fairburn (2008) explicitly assumes that body size is a function of eating disorder diagnosis: "Most patients with bulimia nervosa and eating disorder NOS[1] have a body mass index (BMI) in the healthy range (between 20.0 and 24.9)" (p. 15). He goes on to state that

> by definition, patients with anorexia nervosa are significantly underweight, and this is also true of a proportion of those with eating disorder NOS. At the other end of the weight spectrum, the great majority of patients with binge eating disorder are either overweight or have co-existing obesity (BMI 30 or more) reflecting their general tendency to overeat. (Fairburn, 2008, p. 15)

He also wrote, "Obesity is the general medical disorder most commonly seen among patients with an eating disorder, although the combination is not as common as might be thought because it is largely confined to patients with binge eating disorder" (Fairburn, 2008, p. 253).

It is taken as a given that higher-weight people must be "overeating" and under-reporting food intake—the authors express incredulity that people could possibly be both restricting and at a higher weight. For example, Fairburn (2008) writes, "binge eating apart, overeating is not common among patients with eating disorders, the exception being those with binge eating disorder ... they have a general tendency to overeat" (pp. 14–15). Similarly, he expresses concern that encouraging patients in larger bodies to relax dietary rules could be seen as "endorsing overeating" (Fairburn, 2008, p. 254).

The various CBT manuals express conflicting messages: they state "diets don't work," but continue to emphasize the importance of being in a "healthy weight range." The workbook (Fursland et al., 2007) states, "The goal of weight loss is incompatible with correcting disturbed eating" (Module 5, p. 5), and elsewhere acknowledges that "body weight is under strong physiological control." Despite this, it goes on to recommend that patients should be educated about "healthy ways to lose weight" including "binge-proof dieting," which is "moderate dietary restriction" with "no inherent rules" but "flexible dietary guidelines" (Fairburn, 2008, p. 255). And Waller and colleagues (2007) write that if a patient gains weight the therapist should help "them to accept this weight as the one that they are 'meant to be' (whatever it may be *within the healthy BMI range;*" Waller et al., 2007, p. 171).

Another theme we noted was "It's ok to lose weight—just not now." Waller et al. (2007) write, "Once the eating disorder is less of a pressing issue and food intake is more stable, the focus can then turn to weight loss" and goes on to state "we advise clinicians to take a step back and see the resolution of the eating disorder as the first step in the long process of weight management" (Waller et al. 2007, p. 88).

We also find it problematic that both manuals (Fairburn, 2008; Waller et al., 2007) and a CBT workbook (Fursland et al., 2007) focus on "healthy BMI." Both the CBT manual and workbook give instructions for calculating a client's BMI. The workbook says,

> We live in a society that is weight-obsessed. We don't want you to get too hung up on your weight, but it is useful to know a bit about weight: what you weigh and whether your weight is in the healthy range. It will help you set reasonable goals for yourself. (Module 1, p. 9)

The workbook recommends that clients look up what a "healthy BMI" would be for them and specifies that a BMI over 30 is considered "obese." It also asks clients to journal about their thoughts in response to knowing their BMI.

Another common theme is to predict or promise weight loss once binge eating disorder is successfully treated. This message fails to address the reality that bodies come in all sizes, and it denies the impact of weight stigma. The provider is directed to reassure the patient that if they are in a "normal" BMI category they won't go higher.

> We would like to remind you that most people in the healthy weight range who adopt regular eating end up within 1 kg. of where they started, and some even lose weight. This is because even if you consume more calories than

usual from healthy food choices, you're less likely to binge eat and therefore you'll be ingesting fewer calories. This means you're not actually eating more, you may be eating less, with fewer calories overall. (Fursland et al., 2007, Module 5, page 5)

In CBT, it is common to run behavioral experiments and use the outcome of weight gain to test whether a behavioral change really produces as much weight gain as the patient worries it will cause. For example if a patient holds the belief, "If I eat normal meals, my weight will shoot up," they will be instructed to eat three normal meals and see what happens to their weight over the ensuing weeks. "The process is continued over a number of weeks until the patient learns that the original belief is not accurate and that they can eat three meals a day without significant weight gain" (Waller et al., 2007, p. 219). Unfortunately, this experimental design is stigmatizing: it reinforces the idea sitting at the core—that gaining weight would be a negative consequence, rather than dismantling it.

Could we instead challenge what patients believe will happen if they eat regular meals and or if they gain weight? Exposure can be designed to show them they can tolerate whatever happens. Instead of measuring weight changes we could measure distress, guilt and shame, preoccupation with food and body, or how much time one spends engaging with their eating disorder.

Body image interventions in CBT can also be problematic. Body exposure activities that instruct a patient to face or "expose" their body by wearing more form-fitting or revealing clothing in public fail to properly prepare patients in larger bodies to tolerate an environment that invalidates them. Activities that focus on illustrating to a person that their body image is distorted—and hence, they are "not as fat" as they believe—are also inherently fatphobic.

DBT

DBT as it is written focuses on a combination of acceptance and change. These concepts are not inherently fatphobic, however, their application in practice often is. DBT identifies food as an addictive substance and lists "go on a diet" on a list of recommended pleasurable activities. Providers may recommend weight loss in order to "develop a life worth living" and are encouraged to validate weight concerns of higher weight patients. The book *Dialectical Behavior Therapy for Binge Eating and Bulimia* states therapists should validate the concerns of higher weight patients and "the therapist might add that he or she too worries about the client's weight as the excess pounds reflect an overuse of food to numb or avoid emotions." Additionally, the book states that "reaching a healthy weight is important" (Safer et al., 2009, p. 40).

DBT would require considerable modification to be made fat positive. It is possible to include the core parts of DBT as it was initially created, but the ways that it is practiced—particularly for people with eating disorders—would need to change significantly. Any mention of food as an "addiction" or weight loss as a pleasurable activity or a goal of treatment would need to be removed. The entire manual specific to eating disorders would need to be changed because it is riddled with messages about potential weight loss, body size as a problem, and that individuals of higher weight are eating "too much" or using food to "numb out."

Acceptance and commitment therapy (ACT)

ACT is not inherently weight-biased as initially written; however, its adaptation for the purposes of weight loss is clearly harmful. As with most of the therapies we discuss in this chapter, the motivation behind this adaptation was more likely the revenue opportunity from weight-loss programs than sound psychological practice.

Weight stigma in ACT can manifest in subtle ways. The provider may not identify weight loss as a goal or body size as a problem but goes on to suggest the client's weight is getting in their way and that weight loss would allow them to live a more valued life. ACT is also sometimes used to help the client identify and overcome "barriers" to weight loss.

In order for ACT to be weight-inclusive, all aspects of treatment that focus on weight loss would need to be removed. It is insufficient to remove weight loss recommendations from ACT for eating disorders while in other settings, ACT is specifically being used as a weight loss treatment. We need to entirely remove the harmful idea that higher weight means that someone is going to find less value in their life and that weight loss will allow them to find more of this value.

FBT

FBT for eating disorders tends to exhibit less weight bias than most of the other evidence-based treatments for eating disorders. FBT as developed for anorexia and bulimia discusses weight only as it relates to restoring weight for individuals with anorexia. Although a process for determining goal weights in FBT is not specified in the manual, research shows that clinicians practicing FBT are more likely than providers of other treatment methods to use an individualized approach—the patient's own growth records—rather than a population approach in determining goal weights (Lebow et al., 2018).

The FBT manuals do not go far enough in terms of addressing body diversity by including for example atypical anorexia or weight restoration in any condition other than anorexia. One study on FBT for atypical anorexia demonstrates that there is less focus on weight restoring teens with anorexia who are not in objectively small bodies (Hughes et al., 2017).

General considerations for interventions

Compulsive exercise is a common feature of eating disorders. Most therapies discuss the risks of compulsive or compensatory exercise and recommend limiting or monitoring it. In application, weight bias creeps in: rather than basing a recommendation on the client's symptoms, exercise is often discouraged for those in smaller bodies but encouraged for people in bigger bodies. Specifically, people in higher weight bodies are often encouraged or permitted to continue exercise even when their exercise is clearly compulsive. There are strong cultural messages about the importance of exercise and people in larger bodies are often judged negatively if they do not exercise and often face stigma when they do exercise. They are then blamed or seen as resistant if they do not exercise. DBT talks about the benefits of exercise for enhancing mood. HAES focuses on life-enhancing movement, which is much broader focus.

Another intervention that is common is the use of weighing clients as exposure. The theory is that clients need to be comfortable with their weight as part of their eating disorder recovery and that this happens by being exposed to their weight in treatment using exposure and response prevention.

None of these interventions considers weight stigma when recommending this intervention. They fail to recognize the potential harm or re-traumatization from weighing a higher weight person who has faced stigma regarding their weight throughout their lifetime. They also fail to recognize that these clients will face ongoing stigma at health care appointments such that being comfortable with their weight will not protect them from stigma. Additionally, as discussed previously, many eating disorder providers are weight-biased themselves and may be judging the weight of higher, weight clients. Even if they don't say anything negative to the client about their weight, clients will pick up on this judgment and be harmed.

HAES-aligned treatments

It is crucial for the future of the eating disorder field that we develop HAES-aligned treatments. Even if adaptations to current therapies can align them with HAES, this will take time and even in success, we know that these treatments won't be effective for everybody. Treatment that is HAES-aligned needs to be explicitly fat positive and anti-diet. The treatment needs to state from the start that weight loss will never be a treatment goal. There needs to be a commitment to social justice and acknowledgment of the impact of oppression and marginalization.

The evidence base already exists for HAES. Providing inclusive treatment that is non-stigmatizing is an ethical mandate. Newer treatment models such as Body Trust® that are fully fat positive and weight-inclusive are currently being researched to document their efficacy—but in the meantime, there is no doubt that current therapies as practiced are harming our fat clients. We cannot wait for the creation of a body of literature comparable to the one that exists for current treatments. When we know better, we need to do better. Shifting all treatment to a weight-inclusive, social justice, trauma informed practice will be beneficial for our clients across the weight spectrum.

Revised CBT model

The cognitive model for eating disorders posits that overevaluation of shape and weight drives the entire disorder, and that this fixation is caused by something within the individual, such as low self-esteem. This model fails to address our sociocultural context—society is constantly bombarding individuals with the messages that their worth depends on shrinking their bodies. Individuals in larger bodies face stigma and people of many identities are marginalized. In this context, trying to shrink one's body to retain power and safety is a rational response.

By locating the source of the disorder inside an individual—and failing to acknowledge the external stressors—CBT fails to address these systemic processes. Once we start to acknowledge the role of culture, we can help patients see their struggles as an understandable—if maladaptive—response, rather than a product of pathology or vanity. And we can help them to learn new responses and build resilience. Let's replace the "overevaluation of shape and weight" with "diet culture," and let's replace "significantly low weight" with "suppressed weight" to acknowledge people with anorexia who are not in emaciated bodies. In this way, we can modify the cognitive model to be aligned with HAES.

Trauma informed care

We cannot overstate the importance of trauma informed care. To provide care that is not trauma informed is harmful and unethical. As an eating disorder field, we need to recognize the trauma caused by living in a higher weight body in a world full of weight stigma. Any intervention suggesting weight loss is needed or that being in a higher weight body is wrong will re-traumatize our clients.

Preparing to provide trauma-informed care to all clients with eating disorders includes doing work to unpack our internalized weight stigma. All providers exist in the same weight-biased world as our clients do, and have inevitably internalized weight stigma. If we fail to recognize and address our own weight bias, we will continue to harm our clients. But as we have discussed, these issues are systemic. Attempting to put the field as a whole onto a trauma-informed footing requires the shift not just of individual providers, but of the field's entire structure. Until this happens, our field will be full of landmines for higher weight clients seeking treatment for their eating disorders.

Internalized weight bias as an outcome measure

When research is conducted in the eating disorder field it is rare to see internalized weight bias assessed as a pre and post-treatment measure. We have very little, if any, data on current treatments to indicate whether these models are decreasing or increasing internalized weight bias of clients. In order to give our clients the best chance at ongoing recovery, we need to support them in decreasing internalized weight bias. Given the way current treatment is being utilized and messages delivered in eating disorder treatment, it is possible that many clients are leaving treatment with higher levels of internalized weight bias. All research looking into effectiveness of eating disorder treatments should include internalized weight bias as an outcome measure.

Conclusion

After reviewing the presence of weight stigma in evidence-based psychotherapies for eating disorders and considering what changes would need to be made in order to remove the weight bias, we must ask the question of whether these changes are possible—or whether we need to abandon the current evidence-based practices. Given the exclusion of higher-weight people from the research and the bias in the data, we do not know if the evidence supports these practices for higher weight people. There would also need to be significant edits made to the evidence-based therapies to make them HAES-aligned. Even if this were possible it's unclear how it will happen.

Given that evidence-based treatments are manual-based, manuals would need to be revised and ideally new research completed on the revised approach. This would require dedicated time, money, and commitment on the part of the eating disorder field. If the field is ready to commit to removing weight stigma from treatment approaches, this be possible, however, if the field is not willing to make this commitment, we need to abandon these treatment models.

Note

1 Eating disorder NOS is the diagnosis given to people with clinically significant eating disorders who do not meet criteria for anorexia nervosa or bulimia nervosa. This category has now been renamed Other Specified Feeding or Eating Disorder (OSFED).

References

Bacon, L., & Aphramor, L. (2011). Weight science: Evaluating the evidence for a paradigm shift. *Nutrition Journal*, 10(1), 9. https://doi.org/10.1186/1475-2891-10-9

Brownell, K. D., Puhl, R. M., & Schwartz, M. B., & Rudd, L. (Eds.). (2005). *Weight bias: Nature, consequences, and remedies*. Guilford Publications.

Burgard, D. (2009). What is "Health at Every Size"? In E. Rothblum & S. Solovay (Eds.), *The fat studies reader* (pp. 41–53). New York University Press.

Cooper, Z., Fairburn, C. G., & Hawker, D. M. (2003). *Cognitive-behavioral treatment of obesity: A clinician's guide*. Guilford Press.

Fairburn, C. G. (2008). *Cognitive behavior therapy and eating disorders*. Guilford Press.

Fairburn, C. G., Marcus, M. D., & Wilson, G. T. (1993). Cognitive-behavioral therapy for binge eating and bulimia nervosa: A comprehensive treatment manual. In C. G. Fairburn & G. T. Wilson (Eds.), *Binge eating: Nature, assessment, and treatment* (pp. 361–404). Guilford Press.

Fursland, A., Byrne, S., & Nathan, P. (2007) *Overcoming disordered eating*. Centre for Clinical Interventions.

Hughes, E. K., Le Grange, D., Court, A., & Sawyer, S. M. (2017). A case series of family-based treatment for adolescents with atypical anorexia nervosa. *International Journal of Eating Disorders*, 50(4), 424–432. https://doi.org/10.1002/eat.22662

Lebow, J., Sim, L. A., & Accurso, E. C. (2018). Is there clinical consensus in defining weight restoration for adolescents with anorexia nervosa? *Eating Disorders*, 26(3), 270–277. https://doi.org/10.1080/10640266.2017.1388664

Mann, T., Tomiyama, A. J., Westling, E., Lew, A. M., Samuels, B., & Chatman, J. (2007). Medicare's search for effective obesity treatments: Diets are not the answer. *American Psychologist, 62*(3), 220. https://doi.org/10.1037/0003-066X.62.3.220

Morales, E., & Norcross, J. C. (2010). Evidence-based practices with ethnic minorities: Strange bedfellows no more. *Journal of Clinical Psychology, 66*(8), 821–829. https://doi.org/10.1002/jclp.20712

Neumark-Sztainer, D. (2015). Higher weight status and restrictive eating disorders: An overlooked concern. *Journal of Adolescent Health, 56*(1), 1–2. https://doi.org/10.1016/j.jadohealth.2014.10.261

Neumark-Sztainer, D., Wall, M., Larson, N. I., Eisenberg, M. E., & Loth, K. (2011). Dieting and disordered eating behaviors from adolescence to young adulthood: Findings from a 10-year longitudinal study. *Journal of the American Dietetic Association, 111*(7), 1004–1011. https://doi.org/10.1016/j.jada.2011.04.012

Puhl, R. M., Latner, J. D., King, K. M., & Luedicke, J. (2014). Weight bias among professionals treating eating disorders: Attitudes about treatment and perceived patient outcomes. *International Journal of Eating Disorders, 47*(1), 65–75. https://doi.org/10.1002/eat.22186

Safer, D. L., Telch, C. F., & Chen, E. Y. (2009). *Dialectical behavior therapy for binge eating and bulimia.* Guilford Press.

Stunkard, A. J. (1958). The results of treatment for obesity. *New York State Journal of Medicine, 58*, 79–87.

Waller, G., Cordery, H., Corstorphine, E., Hinrichsen, H., Lawson, R., Mountford, V., & Russell, K. (2007). *Cognitive behavioral therapy for eating disorders: A comprehensive treatment guide.* Cambridge University Press. https://doi.org/10.1017/CBO9781139644204

13 Incorporating fat pedagogy into health care training

Evidence-informed recommendations

Alexandria M. Schmidt and Paula M. Brochu

Weight bias is pervasive and commonly expressed in health care settings and training programs (Brochu et al., 2018; Phelan, Burgess, et al., 2015). For example, in a large survey of first-year medical students, 67% reported negative attitudes toward fat people (Phelan et al., 2014). Over the course of medical school, these negative attitudes worsened from the beginning of first year to the end of fourth year (Phelan, Puhl, et al., 2015). In a large survey of physicians, more than two-thirds viewed "physical inactivity, overeating, and high-fat diet" as primary causes of fatness; more than 50% viewed fat patients as "awkward, unattractive, ugly, and noncompliant," and one-third described their fat patients as "weak-willed, sloppy, or lazy" (Foster et al., 2003, p. 1173). Compounding the problem of weight bias in health care settings, the experience of weight bias itself is a significant stressor that negatively affects health and well-being. For example, perceived weight discrimination increases mortality risk (Sutin et al., 2015) and the development of psychological disorders, such as depression, anxiety, and substance dependence (Hatzenbuehler et al., 2009). Weight bias in health care settings creates a vicious cycle whereby fat people are stigmatized by health care professionals, and in turn avoid seeking treatment in an effort to avoid discrimination (Phelan, Burgess, et al., 2015). This increases the risk for negative health outcomes as a result of inadequate health care due to weight bias.

Systematic training in weight bias is overlooked in health care education. For example, Russell-Mayhew et al. (2016) reviewed primary health care training program curricula in Alberta, Canada. Many of these programs emphasized the health consequences of fatness and highlighted nutrition and lifestyle factors but did not provide education specifically targeting weight bias. In an analysis of textbooks utilized in graduate multicultural courses in psychology, few even acknowledged weight bias (Kasardo, 2019).

In recognition of the problem of weight bias in health care training and among health care professionals, some researchers are examining the efficacy of interventions to reduce weight bias and improve interactions with fat patients. In a review of 17 studies, Alberga et al. (2016) reported a lack of evidence for efficacious weight-stigma reduction interventions among health care professionals. In this chapter, we comprehensively review the efficacy of existing interventions to reduce weight bias among health care professionals and trainees and critically

DOI: 10.4324/9781003057000-15

examine them from the perspective of fat pedagogy (Cameron & Russell, 2016). This is done in an effort to provide evidence-informed recommendations to educators and practitioners that are ethical and weight-inclusive. Fat pedagogy views weight oppression as a serious problem and education as an important intervention (Cameron & Russell, 2016). At its core, fat pedagogy is a radical endeavor to disrupt the status quo: it seeks to increase visibility of interlocking systems of weight oppression and make a positive difference in fat people's lives. Fat pedagogy is built upon basic tenets of size acceptance (Cameron, 2015). In this way, fat pedagogy is distinctly weight-inclusive in recognizing that fatness is not inherently unhealthy, and that weight and health are distinct concepts (Tylka et al., 2014).

A search for peer-reviewed articles that tested interventions designed to reduce weight bias in educational health care settings was conducted using Google Scholar, PubMed, and PsycInfo. To be included in this review, studies must have tested an intervention designed to reduce weight bias among health care trainees or providers and reported statistical analyses that examined whether the intervention was effective in reducing weight bias. Nineteen articles were extracted that met these inclusion criteria. Most of these interventions were conducted with trainees (e.g., medical, kinesiology, dietetics students), though some were conducted with professionals (e.g., nurses, physiotherapists, public health promoters). As such, most of these interventions were conducted in the university or health care setting, though some incorporated service learning experiences outside of the classroom. In reviewing these articles, it became clear that most of the identified interventions did not embrace fat pedagogy and actually reinforced aspects of weight stigma, even though they were designed with the intention of reducing weight bias.

Six primary types of weight bias reduction intervention were identified: "obesity" curriculum, weight bias awareness, controllability, contact, empathy, and multi-component interventions. "Obesity" curriculum interventions focus on increasing medical knowledge about fatness (Gayer et al., 2011). Weight bias awareness interventions provide information to increase awareness of weight bias and its consequences (e.g., McVey et al., 2013). Controllability interventions provide information on the uncontrollable reasons for fatness, such as genetics, environment, and stressors, to reduce attributions of responsibility and blame (e.g., O'Brien et al., 2010). Contact interventions provide interaction experiences with fat patients (e.g., Kushner et al., 2014). Empathy interventions encourage perspective-taking and imagining the life and experience of fat people (e.g., Matharu et al., 2014). Finally, multi-component interventions utilize more than one strategy to reduce weight bias (e.g., Rukavina et al., 2010). Each of these interventions is described below; many of them were informed by biomedical, weight-normative approaches to health and as a result are quite stigmatizing.

"Obesity" curriculum

One of the articles identified in this review tested an "obesity" curriculum. Gayer et al. (2011) proposed that increasing comprehensive medical knowledge about fatness would decrease weight bias. The curriculum covered topics such as epidemiology, weight management interventions, and chronic diseases associated with fatness. This curriculum was provided to medical students over 4 years of medical school and included class programming, assessment of knowledge, and virtual patient case presentations. The curriculum increased students' medical knowledge and decreased negative stereotyping of fat people, which was sustained throughout all 4 years of medical school. This intervention provided students with a traditional, weight-normative, biomedical perspective on fatness that was focused on addressing the so-called "obesity" epidemic. Weight bias was not included in the curriculum.

Weight bias awareness

Three of the articles identified in this review tested interventions designed to increase awareness of weight bias. These interventions ranged from sensitivity training on how to treat fat patients respectfully and ethically, to the provision of information on the pervasiveness and harm of weight bias and ways in which weight bias could be reduced in practice. Gujral et al. (2011) compared two hospitals, one that provided bariatric sensitivity training and one that did not, and found that nurses in the hospital that offered the training reported more positive attitudes toward fat people. However, their beliefs regarding the controllability of weight did not differ from the nurses in the hospital that did not offer the training. Barra and Singh Hernandez (2018) provided nursing students with "obesity" sensitivity training and found that more positive attitudes toward fat people were reported at the end of the 15-week training. McVey et al. (2013) provided public health promoters with a full-day professional development workshop on weight bias awareness. Participants reported decreases in anti-fat attitudes and internalization of the thin ideal, and increases in self-efficacy to address weight bias, that were maintained 6 weeks later.

These findings indicate that weight bias may be reduced by mere awareness-raising. However, it is important to note that these interventions sent participants conflicting messages that simultaneously described the harm of weight bias while maintaining that fatness is unhealthy. In this way, weight bias awareness was predominantly framed as an important strategy to reduce the negative health consequences of fatness. No attempts were made to increase understanding of interlocking systems of fat oppression, with relatively little emphasis on providing ethical and respectful care to all patients (but see Barra & Singh Hernandez, 2018). Instead, most of these interventions were focused on "obesity" prevention, weight management, and "healthy weight" promotion.

Controllability

Two of the articles identified in this review tested interventions with students that focused on weakening belief in the controllability of weight in an effort to reduce blame and responsibility placed on fat people. Persky and Eccleston (2011) randomly assigned medical students to one of three conditions that provided information on the role of genetics in fatness, the role of behavior in fatness, or an unrelated medical condition (chronic headache pain; control). After learning this information from a short, scientific article, participants interacted with a fat virtual patient presenting for her annual exam. Participants in the genetic condition attributed a greater percentage of body weight to genetics, held the patient less responsible for her weight, stereotyped the patient less, and recommended weight loss, diet, and exercise consultation less frequently. The researchers discussed these findings as a double-edged sword; although information highlighting the genetic contribution to fatness decreased weight stigmatization of the patient, it also decreased the provision of health behavior recommendations. From a fat pedagogical perspective, however, these results would be viewed as a success, as weight loss recommendations are viewed as unethical and harmful (Rothblum, 2018; Tylka et al., 2014).

O'Brien et al. (2010) randomly assigned students to one of three course sections that taught controllable reasons for fatness that emphasized personal responsibility and control, uncontrollable reasons for fatness that emphasized genetics and environmental factors, or alcohol use (control condition) over 5 weeks. They found that participants in the uncontrollable condition demonstrated less negative implicit weight attitudes and stereotypes after the intervention and reported weaker belief in the role of willpower and control in dieting. However, there were no changes in explicit anti-fat attitudes or belief in the controllability of weight. In this study, even participants in the uncontrollable condition were presented with information from the dominant, biomedical paradigm that equates fatness with poor health (i.e., the prevalence and health consequences of fatness), and, as such, stigmatized fatness even though its goal was to reduce weight bias.

Contact

Three of the articles identified in this review examined the role of contact with fat patients in weight bias reduction. In a large study of medical students, Meadows, Higgs, et al. (2017) found that students who had more positive contact experiences with fat patients during medical school reported more positive attitudes toward treating fat patients. The quality of the contact is what mattered; the frequency of contact with fat patients did not influence participants' attitudes. However, participants' self-reported their frequency and favorability of contact with fat patients during medical school; the effects of a contact-driven intervention were not directly tested. Roberts et al. (2011) paired medical students with a fat patient undergoing bariatric surgery, in which they established a longitudinal patient relationship over the course of a year. Only 4 out of 13 students self-selected into this elective program. Nevertheless, the contact intervention improved attitudes toward fat patients and fatness. However, some anti-fat attitudes and beliefs remained, most likely due to the training received, such as believing it necessary to educate fat patients about weight-related health risks and recommend surgical evaluations for fat patients.

Kushner et al. (2014) designed an intervention in which medical students read articles about weight stigma and patient communication, and then engaged in a structured encounter with a fat standardized patient. After the intervention, students reported decrease in negative weight stereotyping and increase in empathy and counseling confidence; 1 year later, the endorsement of negative weight stereotypes reverted to baseline, although the improvements in empathy and confidence were maintained. As with most of the interventions reviewed in this chapter, from a fat pedagogical perspective, the implementation of this intervention is inherently problematic. The scenarios enacted by the standardized patients were primarily focused on weight loss and framed the patient's weight as a medical problem. Accordingly, the communication strategies taught to students focused on weight counseling, such as how to initiate conversations about weight with fat patients and encourage weight loss.

Empathy

Three of the articles included this review tested empathy induction as an intervention to reduce weight bias among health care trainees. In addition to measuring contact, Meadows, Higgs, et al. (2017) also asked medical students how many empathy training hours they received during medical school (i.e., seeing things from the patient's perspective). Overall, they found that hours of empathy training did not predict attitudes toward fat patients. However, this varied by student; students who initially reported more egalitarianism, cognitive and emotional empathy, and comfort with uncertainty, reported less negative attitudes toward fat patients the more empathy training they reported receiving. It is unknown whether any of the empathy training students received was focused on empathizing with fat patients specifically.

The remaining articles utilized experiential learning to increase empathy toward fat patients. Matharu et al. (2014) randomly assigned medical students to a play-reading that featured fat women's discrimination experiences set in a liposuction clinic, or a standard lecture on "obesity" management. Students who participated in the dramatic reading reported less negative anti-fat attitudes and more patient-centered care (rather than prescriptive care management) than students who attended the lecture. Empathy increased for both conditions. By contrast, Cotugna and Mallick (2010) had dietetics students follow a calorie-restricted diet for 1 week in a nutrition elective course to better understand and empathize with fat people and the struggle to lose weight. All students in the course were required to participate for a class assignment; they were not screened for pre-existing eating disorder symptoms or history. The researchers reported a significant change in anti-fat stereotyping, but the direction of the change was not clear and descriptive statistics were not reported. The researchers described the dieting intervention as "an effective and simple tool that educators can easily implement in a classroom setting to help prepare dietetics and other health care students to deal with the ever growing obesity epidemic" (p. 324). From a fat pedagogical perspective, this intervention is unethical, disrespectful, and harmful, as it encourages dieting, emphasizes weight loss, and reduces the fat experience to a 1-week diet. The intervention may have caused a relapse for students with eating disorder history and reinforced unhealthy dieting behaviors for students who experienced weight stigma, body image concerns, or disordered relationships with food.

Multi-component

Eight of the articles identified in this review tested multi-component interventions in which more than one strategy was incorporated in the intervention, making it impossible to disentangle the effects of each intervention type. Jones and Forhan (2021) conducted a day-long educational seminar with physiotherapists on how to work effectively and sensitively with fat patients undergoing joint replacement. In addition to providing information to increase weight bias awareness, information on the complexity of fatness was also provided. Although the training weakened participants' weight control beliefs, more negative attitudes toward fat people were reported after the training. The seminar was led by clinicians and researchers with expertise in bariatrics and joint replacement, who focus on "obesity" prevention and weight management.

Rukavina et al. (2008, 2010) conducted interventions with kinesiology students in a measurement and testing course that incorporated weight bias awareness, controllability attributions, and empathy induction over a period of 6 weeks. The intervention included classroom components and a service learning project in which students administered fitness tests to elementary-aged children and then reflected on their experience. Students reported weaker weight control/ blame beliefs after the interventions; in the 2010 study, students also reported less social/character disparagement of fat people. However, reports of anti-fat stereotyping and fat people's romantic/physical attractiveness did not change, nor did students' implicit attitudes and stereotypes. Care must be taken to ensure that interventions that incorporate service learning do not unwittingly stigmatize fatness, reinforce weight stereotypes, or leave students without the tools necessary to effectively and ethically manage the experience in which they are placed.

Poustchi et al. (2013) and Swift et al. (2013) showed videos to medical students about weight bias that increased weight bias awareness, addressed controllability, induced empathy, and debunked weight stereotypes. These videos were developed by the Rudd Center for Food Policy and Obesity. Poustchi et al. (2013) found that participants reported weaker weight controllability beliefs and endorsed weight stereotypes less strongly after watching the video and engaging in class discussion, although their attitudes toward fat people did not change. Swift et al. (2013) found that endorsement of negative weight attitudes, stereotypes, and weight control beliefs decreased immediately after watching the videos, although only the change in weight control beliefs was maintained 6 weeks later. Although focused on weight bias, these videos were developed from a weight-normative perspective on health.

Wiese et al. (1992) and Wijayatunga et al. (2019) conducted classroom-based interventions in which they randomly assigned medical students and kinesiology students, respectively, to one of two course sections that incorporated weight bias awareness, controllability attributions, and empathy induction, or provided standard programming. Lecture, videos, and group activities were utilized. Wiese et al. (1992) found that students in the intervention reported greater belief in the genetic contribution to fatness, reduced blame of fat people, and less negative weight stereotyping; 1 year later, students continued to rate the importance of genetic factors and blame fat people less. Similarly, Wijayatunga et al. (2019) found that weight control/blame beliefs decreased among students in the intervention and were maintained 1 month later. However, explicit anti-fat attitudes did not change. Implicit attitudes worsened among students in the control condition, highlighting the harm of traditional "obesity" curricula. Although both of these studies presented some elements of critical weight science to learners, the interventions were ultimately framed from a weight-normative perspective that views fatness as a problem.

Brochu (2020) conducted a weight bias seminar with clinical psychology trainees that provided information on critical weight science that challenged common assumptions about weight and health, including the controllability of weight. The seminar also provided information on the prevalence and harm of weight bias. Weight-inclusive models of health such as Health at Every Size (HAES™) were introduced to trainees. Participants reported weaker weight controllability beliefs, anti-fat attitudes, and negative attitudes toward fat clients 1 week after the training. Furthermore, controllability beliefs mediated the effect of the intervention on overall and client-specific anti-fat attitudes. Informing trainees of critical weight science and weight-inclusive models of health encourages a social-justice oriented perspective to understand the complexity of fatness. It also supports a shift in focus from weight and weight loss to health and well-being for people of all sizes. However, although the seminar emphasized respectful and ethical care for all people, the focus on health may morph weight bias into healthism for some students and require additional intervention.

Recommendations

Each of the interventions identified in this review showed efficacy in reducing some aspect of weight bias among health care professionals and trainees. These findings, however, were neither consistent across studies nor consistent within most studies across measures. Furthermore, any improvements that were obtained were not necessarily maintained over time. There is well-founded concern that any gains made by such interventions may be countered by exposure to weight bias in other training and health care settings; intensive and extensive education programming is recommended, including booster sessions and ongoing support to maintain intervention efficacy (e.g., Gayer et al., 2011; McVey et al., 2013; O'Brien et al., 2010). It remains unclear whether improvement in weight-based attitudes and beliefs influence the behavior of health care practitioners in terms of patient care and other clinically-relevant outcomes.

Perhaps most importantly for the purpose of this review, the vast majority of the interventions were influenced by the dominant, weight-normative paradigm that inherently stigmatizes fatness by viewing it as a disease or medical problem. Only one of the studies mentioned fat pedagogy (Brochu, 2020), and few mentioned weight-inclusive models of health or the concept of HAES (Brochu, 2020; McVey et al., 2013; Rukavina et al., 2008). In addition, few recommended a patient-centered care approach, such as addressing weight only when solicited by the patient first (Barra & Singh Hernandez, 2018; Matharu et al., 2014). From a fat pedagogical perspective, this is concerning because there are few studies that provide recommendations that are both evidence-informed and ethically-sound.

There are serious ethical concerns with some of the interventions, particularly those that were motivated to improve communication with fat patients regarding weight-loss counseling or address the so-called "obesity" epidemic (e.g., Gayer et al., 2011; Kushner et al., 2014). Alarmingly, Cotugna and Mallick (2010) required dietetics students to follow a calorie-restricted diet to "increase sensitivity and reduce existing biases" (p. 321). For the past several decades, the research is clear that not only are diets ineffective for weight loss over the long-term, they harm physical and psychological health and well-being (Rothblum, 2018). In reviewing the literature, other interventions that did not meet our inclusion criteria also raised serious ethical concerns. These interventions utilized experiential methods to simulate fatness, such as having health care professionals or standardized patients wear fat suits (Hales et al., 2018; Herrmann-Werner et al., 2019). The experience of fatness and weight bias are not represented when a thin person wears a fat suit; these simulations reduce the experience of a fat person as uncomfortable, embarrassing, and even immobilizing (Meadows, Daníeldóttir, et al., 2017). The education and research practice of fat simulation suits fundamentally violates values of body equality and social justice.

Most of the interventions were underpinned by sentiments that perpetuate weight stigma. The implementation of the interventions emphasized the prevalence of high body mass indices, the health consequences of fatness, and health care costs. Many of the interventions framed fatness as problem that is devastating to both fat people and health care systems (e.g., Roberts et al., 2011). This likely limited the effectiveness of the interventions. Few interventions informed students of alternative models of health that did not stigmatize fatness (e.g., Brochu, 2020). Considering that people learn a great deal from subtle societal messages without even realizing it, unlearning this information must be done consciously and intentionally. As such, interventions must directly address misconceptions regarding weight and health, debunk stereotypes of fat people, and raise awareness of weight bias. This can be accomplished by providing information on critical weight science and weight-inclusive models of health, focusing on well-being rather than weight loss, and adopting a social-justice orientation (Bacon & Aphramor, 2011; Logel et al., 2015; Nutter et al., 2016; Tylka et al., 2014).

Perhaps the most effective interventions incorporate multiple components in combination with one another, filling in gaps that single intervention strategies might miss. For example, "obesity" curricula neglect raising awareness of weight bias, whereas empathy interventions may overlook controllability attributions, and contact interventions may not raise awareness of critical weight science or weight bias. For the health care educator interested in incorporating fat pedagogy into their curricula, the following questions must also be considered: Is the intervention bringing awareness to the problems of focusing on weight or weight loss? Are alternative health approaches presented that are weight-inclusive, well-being centered, and social-justice oriented? Does the intervention avoid language and procedures that perpetuate weight bias? Is the intervention isolated, or taking place in a bubble where the weight-normative status quo is otherwise maintained? The process of fat pedagogy continually evolves (Cameron & Russell, 2016). It requires dedication to thoughtful self-reflection and commitment to personal growth. Fat pedagogy educators seek to compassionately meet learners where they are, while striving to create meaningful change to improve the lives of fat people. When incorporating fat pedagogy into health care training, nothing less will do.

References

*Articles included in review.

Alberga, A. S., Pickering, B. J., Hayden, K. A., Ball, G. D. C., Edwards, A., Jelinski, S., Nutter, S., Oddie, S., Sharma, A. M., & Russell-Mayhew, S. (2016). Weight bias reduction in health professionals: A systematic review. *Clinical Obesity*, 6(3), 175–188. https://doi.org/10.1111/cob.12147

Bacon, L., & Aphramor, L. (2011). Weight science: Evaluating the evidence for a paradigm shift. *Nutrition Journal*, 10(1), Article 9. https://doi.org/10.1186/1475-2891-10-9

*Barra, M., & Singh Hernandez, S. S. (2018). Too big to be seen: Weight-based discrimination among nursing students. *Nursing Forum*, 53(4), 529–534. https://doi.org/10.1111/nuf.12282

*Brochu, P. M. (2020). Testing the effectiveness of a weight bias educational intervention among psychology trainees. *Journal of Applied Social Psychology*. Advance online publication. https://doi.org/10.1111/jasp.12653

Brochu, P. M., Pearl, R. L., & Simontacchi, L. A. (2018). Weight stigma and related social factors in psychological care. In S. Cassin, R. Hawa, & S. Sockalingham (Eds.), *Psychological care in severe obesity: A practical and integrated approach* (pp. 42–60). Cambridge University Press. https://doi.org/10.1017/9781108241687.004

Cameron, E. (2015). Teaching resources for post-secondary educators who challenge dominant "obesity" discourse. *Fat Studies*, 4(2), 212–226. https://doi.org/10.1080/21604851.2015.998977

Cameron, E., & Russell, C. (Eds.). (2016). *The fat pedagogy reader: Challenging weight-based oppression through critical education*. Peter Lang.

*Cotugna, N., & Mallick, A. (2010). Following a calorie-restricted diet may help in reducing healthcare students' fat-phobia. *Journal of Community Health*, 35(3), 321–324. https://doi.org/10.1007/s10900-010-9226-9

Foster, G. D., Wadden, T. A., Makris, A. P., Davidson, D., Sanderson, R. S., Allison, D. B., & Kessler, A. (2003). Primary care physicians' attitudes about obesity and its treatment. *Obesity Research*, 11(10), 1168–1177. https://doi.org/10.1038/oby.2003.161

*Gayer, G. G., Weiss, J., & Clearfield, M. (2011). Fundamentals for an osteopathic obesity designed study: The effects of education on osteopathic medical students' attitudes regarding obesity. *Journal of the American Osteopathic Association*, 117(8), 495–502. https://doi.org/10.7556/jaoa.2017.099

Gujral, H., Tea, C., & Sheridan, M. (2011). Evaluation of nurse's attitudes toward adult patients of size. *Surgery for Obesity and Related Diseases, 7*(4), 536–540. https://doi. org/10.1016/j.soard.2011.03.008

Hales, C., Gray, L., Russel, L., & MacDonald, C. (2018). A qualitative study to explore the impact of simulating extreme obesity on health care professionals' attitudes and perceptions. *Ostomy Wound Management, 64*(1), 18–24. https://doi.org/10.25270/owm.2018.1.1824

Hatzenbuehler, M. L., Keyes, K. M., & Hasin, D. S. (2009). Associations between perceived weight discrimination and the prevalence of psychiatric disorders in the general population. *Obesity, 17*, 2033–2039. https://doi.org/10.1038/oby.2009.131

Herrmann-Werner, A., Loda, T., Wiesner, L. M., Erschens, R. S., Junne, F., & Zipfel, S. (2019). Is an obesity simulation suit in an undergraduate medical communication class a valuable teaching tool? A cross-sectional proof of concept study. *BMJ Open, 9*(8), e029738. https://doi.org/10.1136/bmjopen-2019-029738

Jones, C. A., & Forhan, M. (2021). Addressing weight bias and stigma of obesity amongst physiotherapists. *Physiotherapy Theory and Practice, 37*(7), 808–816. https://doi.org/10.1 080/09593985.2019.1648623

Kasardo, A. E. (2019). Size as diversity absent from multicultural textbooks. *Women & Therapy, 42*(1–2), 181–190. https://doi.org/10.1080/02703149.2018.1524069

*Kushner, R. F., Zeiss, D. M., Feinglass, J. M., & Yelen, M. (2014). An obesity educational intervention for medical students addressing weight bias and communication skills using standardized patients. *BMC Medical Education, 14*(1), Article 53. https://doi. org/10.1186/1472-6920-14-53

Logel, C., Stinson, D. A., & Brochu, P. M. (2015). Weight loss is not the answer: A well-being solution to the "obesity problem." *Social and Personality Psychology Compass, 9*(12), 678–695. https://doi.org/10.1111/spc3.12223

*Matharu, K., Shapiro, J. F., Hammer, R. R., Kravitz, R. L., Wilson, M. D., & Fitzgerald, F. T. (2014). Reducing obesity prejudice in medical education. *Education for Health, 27*(3), 231–237. https://doi.org/10.4103/1357-6283.152176

*McVey, G. L., Walker, K. S., Beyers, J., Harrison, H. L., Simkins, S. W., & Russell-Mayhew, S. (2013). Integrating weight bias awareness and mental health promotion into obesity prevention delivery: A public health pilot study. *Preventing Chronic Disease, 10*, Article 120185. https://doi.org/10.5888/pcd10.120185

Meadows, A., Danielsdóttir, S., Calogero, R., & O'Reilly, C. (2017). Why fat suits do not advance the scientific study of weight stigma. *Obesity, 25*(2), 275. https://doi. org/10.1002/oby.21742

*Meadows, A., Higgs, S., Burke, S. E., Dovido, J. F., van Ryn, M., & Phelan, S. M. (2017). Social dominance orientation, dispositional empathy, and need for cognitive closure moderate the impact of empathy-skills training, but not patient contact, on medical students' negative attitudes toward higher-weight patients. *Frontiers in Psychology, 8*, Article 504. https://doi.org/10.3389/fpsyg.2017.00504

Nutter, S., Russell-Mayhew, S., Alberga, A. S., Arthur, N., Kassan, A., Lund, D. E., Sesma-Vazquez, M., & Williams, E. (2016). Positioning of weight bias: Moving towards social justice. *Journal of Obesity, 2016*, Article 3753650. https://doi.org/10.1155/2016/3753650

*O'Brien, K. S., Puhl, R. M., Latner, J. D., Mir, A. S., & Hunter, J. A. (2010). Reducing anti-fat prejudice in preservice health students: A randomized controlled trial. *Obesity, 18*(11), 2318–2144. https://doi.org/10.1038/oby.2010.79

*Persky, S., & Eccleston, C. P. (2011). Impact of genetic causal information on medical students' clinical encounters with an obese virtual patient: Health promotion and social stigma. *Annals of Behavior Medicine, 41*(3), 363–372. https://doi.org/10.1007/s12160-010-9242-0

Phelan, S. M., Dovidio, J. F., Puhl, R. M., Burgess, D. J., Nelson, D. B., Yeazel, M. W., Hardeman, R., Perry, S., & van Ryn, M. (2014). Implicit and explicit weight bias in a national sample of 4,732 medical students: The medical student CHANGES study. *Obesity, 22*(4), 1201–1208. https://doi.org/10.1002/oby.20687

Phelan, S. M., Burgess, D. J., Yeazel, M. W., Hellerstedt, W. L., Griffin, J. M., & van Ryn, M. (2015). Impact of weight bias and stigma on quality of care and outcomes for patients with obesity. *Obesity Reviews, 16*(4), 319–326. https://doi.org/10.1111/obr.12266

Phelan, S. M., Puhl, R. M., Burke, S. E., Hardeman, R., Dovidio, J. F., Nelson, D. B., Przedworski, J., Burgess, D. M., Perry, S., Yeazel, M. W., & van Ryn, M. (2015). The mixed impact of medical school on medical students' implicit and explicit weight bias. *Medical Education, 49*(10), 983–992. https://doi.org/10.1111/medu.12770

*Poustchi, Y., Saks, N. S., Piasecki, A. K., Hahn, K. A., & Ferrante, J. M. (2013). Brief intervention effective in reducing weight bias in medical students. *Family Medicine, 45*(5), 345–348.

*Roberts, D. H., Kane, E. M., Jones, D. B., Almeida, J. M., Bell, S. K., Weinstiein, A. R., & Schwartzstein, R. M. (2011). Teaching medical students about obesity: A pilot program to address an unmet need through longitudinal relationships with bariatric surgery patients. *Surgical Innovation, 18*(2), 176–183. https://doi.org/10.1177/1553350611399298

Rothblum, E. D. (2018). Slim chance for permanent weight loss. *Archives of Scientific Psychology, 6*(1), 63–69. https://doi.org/10.1037/arc0000043

*Rukavina, P. B., Li, W., & Rowell, M. B. (2008). A service learning based intervention to change attitudes toward obese individuals in kinesiology pre-professionals. *Social Psychology of Education, 11*(1), 95–112. https://doi.org/10.1007/s11218-007-9039-6

*Rukavina, P. B., Li, W., Shen, B., & Sun, H. (2010). A service learning based project to change implicit and explicit bias toward obese individuals in kinesiology pre-professionals. *Obesity Facts, 3*(2), 117–126. https://doi.org/10.1159/000302794

Russell-Mayhew, S., Nutter, S., Alberga, A., Jelinski, S., Ball, G. D. C., Edwards, A., Oddie, S., Sharma, A. M., Pickering, B., & Forhan, M. (2016). Environmental scan of weight bias exposure in primary health care training programs. *Canadian Journal for the Scholarship of Teaching and Learning, 7*(2), Article 5. https://doi.org/10.5206/cjsotl-rcacea.2016.2.5

Sutin, A. R., Stephan, Y., & Terracciano, A. (2015). Weight discrimination and mortality. *Psychological Science, 26*(11), 1803–1811. https://doi.org/10.1177/0956797615601103

*Swift, J. A., Tischler, V., Markham, S., Gunning, I., Glazebrook, C., Beer, C., & Puhl, R. (2013). Are anti-stigma films a useful strategy for reducing weight bias among trainee healthcare professionals? Results of a pilot randomized control trial. *Obesity Facts, 6*(1), 91–102. https://doi.org/10.1159/000348714

Tylka, T. L., Annunziato, R. A., Burgard, D., Daníelsdóttir, S., Shuman, E., Davis, C., & Calogero, R. M. (2014). The weight-inclusive versus weight-normative approach to health: Evaluating the evidence for prioritizing well-being over weight loss. *Journal of Obesity, 2014.* Article 983495. https://doi.org/10.1155/2014/983495

*Wiese, H. J. C., Wilson, J. F., Jones, R. A., & Neises, M. (1992). Obesity stigma reduction in medical students. *International Journal of Obesity, 16*, 859–868.

*Wijayatunga, N. N., Kim, Y., Butsch, W. S., & Dhurandhar, E. J. (2019). The effects of a teaching intervention on weight bias among kinesiology undergraduate students. *International Journal of Obesity, 43*(11), 2273–2281. https://doi.org/10.1038/s41366-019-0325-0

14 Applying the attribution-value model of prejudice to fat pedagogy in health care settings

Paula M. Brochu and Roya Amirniroumand

There is a need for weight bias to be effectively addressed in health care training programs. Health care professionals often report negative attitudes and stereotypes about fat people, reducing the quality of health care provision (Brochu et al., 2018; Phelan et al., 2015). Some researchers have begun testing interventions to reduce weight bias in health care training settings, with limited success (Alberga et al., 2016). In general, research shows inconsistent outcomes of such interventions for weight bias reduction (Daníelsdóttir et al., 2010; Lee et al., 2014). One mechanism that underlies weight bias is weight controllability beliefs (Crandall, 1994). Interventions that seek to change people's beliefs about the causes of weight and the ability to control body weight are known as controllability interventions. In this chapter, a critical analysis of weight bias reduction interventions that focus on changing controllability beliefs is conducted from the perspective of the attribution-value model of prejudice (Crandall et al., 2001). This analysis is conducted in order to better understand the mechanisms underlying the effective incorporation of fat pedagogy (Cameron & Russell, 2016) in health care training programs.

Attribution-value model of prejudice

The attribution-value model of prejudice is a general model of prejudice that identifies two interrelated factors that increase prejudice toward social groups: attributions of controllability and cultural value (Crandall et al., 2001). Attribution theory argues that social bias is shaped by people's perceptions of controllability, responsibility, and blame over a stereotyped characteristic (Weiner, 1995; Weiner et al., 1988). Cultural value refers to the social ideologies that lead people to perceive particular social groups negatively, for example by perceiving a social group as lazy or lacking intelligence (Crandall et al., 2001). Applied to weight bias, prejudice is exacerbated when fat people are attributed responsibility for their weight, and when fatness is negatively culturally valued. The attribution-value model of prejudice has been supported in cross-cultural studies, with more pronounced effects in individualistic cultures (Crandall et al., 2001; Crandall & Martinez, 1996).

The attribution-value model of prejudice may offer some insight into the mixed outcomes of controllability interventions designed to reduce weight bias. The

DOI: 10.4324/9781003057000-16

model implies that, in order to be effective, weight bias reduction interventions must reduce weight controllability beliefs as well as challenge the notion that fat is bad. For the most part, controllability interventions focus on the attribution aspect without addressing the value component. Indeed, many controllability interventions frame fatness as a public health crisis to participants (e.g., O'Brien et al., 2010). This approach may, in fact, promote and perpetuate stigma. Specifically, controllability-based weight-bias reduction interventions applied in health care training settings may be limited depending on whether the information is perceived as believable by participants (i.e., whether people's controllability attributions about weight actually change), and whether the broader social context of the intervention portrays fat as bad (e.g., interventions that are weight-loss centered or focus on the prevalence and consequences of fatness).

A critical analysis of controllability interventions

Let us first consider two research examples of controllability interventions conducted with convenience samples. As one example, Teachman et al. (2003) randomly assigned participants recruited at the beach to one of three conditions in which they read a brief article about the role of genetics or behavior in fatness, or a no-information control condition. They found that participants in the genetic condition were as likely to believe that body weight is under personal control as participants in the control condition. Thus, the information presented was not believed by participants, and unsurprisingly, the intervention did not reduce weight bias. As another example, Lippa and Sanderson (2012) randomly assigned online participants to one of three conditions in which they read information about (a) the causal role of genetics in fatness, (b) the causal role of the environment in fatness, or (c) a gene-environment interaction. In addition, all participants read an excerpt that focused on the increasing prevalence of fatness as a major public health concern because it is associated with negative physical health outcomes. Even though participants in this study who read information about the role of genetics in fatness reported weaker weight controllability beliefs, this did not generalize to their weight-related attitudes, which did not change and remained negative. Thus, if the goal is to reduce weight bias, it is important that controllability interventions do not inadvertently reinforce a negative cultural value of fatness.

Schmidt and Brochu (this book) identified 10 interventions designed to reduce weight bias among health care professionals or trainees that addressed controllability attributions and measured weight control beliefs. In the present chapter, each controllability intervention designed to reduce weight bias will be critically examined from the theoretical lens of the attribution-value model of prejudice. Of these 10 interventions, nine might be considered failures and one might be considered successful from the perspective of the attribution-value model.

The strategies utilized in these controllability interventions range from having health care professionals read research articles about the role of genetics as a mechanism underlying fatness (Persky & Eccleston, 2011), watch videos about weight bias and discrimination such as the University of Connecticut Rudd Center's (2009a, 2009b) "Weight Prejudice: Myths & Facts" and "Weight Bias in Healthcare" (Poutschi et al., 2013; Swift et al., 2013), and attend class lectures or workshops that range from a single session to several (Brochu, 2020; Jones & Forhan, 2019; O'Brien et al., 2010; Rukavina et al., 2008, 2010; Wiese et al., 1992; Wijayatunga et al., 2019). Some interventions incorporated service learning or other experiential activities such as conducting fitness tests of elementary-aged school children (Rukavina et al., 2008, 2010) and interacting with a fat virtual patient (Persky & Eccleston, 2011). Despite the diversity in the mode of the controllability intervention, the primary goal driving each of these interventions is to reduce attendees' perceptions that weight status is entirely within a person's control. Some interventions do this by emphasizing the role of uncontrollable causes for fatness, such as genetics and the environment (O'Brien et al., 2010; Persky & Eccelston, 2011; Wiese et al., 1992; Wijayatunga et al., 2019). Other interventions do this by challenging stereotypes that fat people eat too much or engage in too little physical activity; for example, Wiese et al. (1992) communicated to medical students in their intervention that, contrary to popular thought, there are no differences in calorie intake between people based on their body size. Yet other interventions do this by communicating to attendees the complexity of weight and fatness and how it is not solely determined by a single controllable or behavioral factor (Jones & Forhan, 2019).

Weight controllability beliefs

First, the good news. Each of the 10 controllability interventions was effective in reducing health care professionals' and trainees' weight controllability beliefs. These interventions were effective in changing current and future health care workers' attributions regarding the controllability of weight. For example, participants less strongly endorsed items such as "Fat people tend to be fat pretty much through their own fault" from the Willpower subscale of Crandall's (1994) Anti-Fat Attitudes Questionnaire after participating in these controllability interventions in health care education and training settings. Evidence suggests that these decreases in endorsement of weight controllability beliefs persisted and were maintained over time in studies that utilized longitudinal, follow-up designs. Specifically, Wijayatunga et al. (2019) found that the reduction in beliefs holding fat people responsible for their weight and blaming them persisted over a period of 1 month among a sample of kinesiology pre-professionals. Similarly, Swift et al. (2013) found that the reduction in weight controllability beliefs persisted over a period of 6 weeks among a sample of dietician and medical students. Notably, Wiese et al. (1992) found that medical students continued to blame fat people less for their weight 1 year after the intervention. However, even though all of the studies were effective in reducing participants' weight-control beliefs, studies varied in the extent of this success. For example, Persky and Eccleston (2011) reported that 31% of medical students in the genetic condition, and 20% of medical students in the behavioral condition, did not believe the premise of the article they read about the genetic or behavioral causes of fatness. Each of these participants instead endorsed the view that fatness is the outcome of an interaction between both genetics and behavior. Nevertheless, participants in the genetic condition reported that a greater percentage of body weight was due to genetics and held the fat virtual patient that they interacted with as less responsible for her weight, than participants in the behavioral condition. Thus, in general, researchers have a solid understanding of how to change people's attributions about the controllability of weight and application of this knowledge in health care education and training settings has been largely successful.

Weight stereotypes and attitudes

Now for the bad news. Although each of these controllability interventions presented to health care professionals or trainees was effective in reducing weight controllability beliefs, they showed mixed effectiveness in reducing participants' endorsement of negative weight stereotypes and attitudes. Only four studies demonstrated some effectiveness in reducing weight stereotypes. In Wiese et al.'s (1992) intervention, medical students who learned about genetic contributions to weight status continued to less strongly endorse negative weight stereotypes 1 year after the intervention (i.e., lazy, sloppy, dull, lacking self-control). Participants exposed to information about the genetic mechanisms underlying weight also reported less weight stereotyping of the fat virtual patient in Persky and Eccleston's (2011) study. Poutschi et al. (2013) and Swift et al. (2013) showed that participants less strongly endorsed weight stereotypes after watching a video-based intervention, though in Swift et al.'s study weight stereotyping returned to baseline levels 6 weeks later. Other studies, however, did not lead to changes in weight stereotyping. For example, O'Brien et al.'s (2010) lecture-based intervention over 5 weeks about uncontrollable reasons for weight among preservice health students did not change participants' implicit stereotyping of fat people. However, there is some evidence that the intervention protected against students' implicit stereotypes worsening over time, as participants who learned about controllable reasons for weight showed more negative implicit weight stereotyping at posttest. Finally, Rukavina et al.'s (2008, 2010) classroom and service learning-based interventions did not change kinesiology pre-professionals' endorsement of weight stereotypes. Thus, whereas some studies that were effective in reducing participants' beliefs regarding the controllability of weight were also effective in reducing participants' endorsement of negative weight stereotypes, others were not.

Similar mixed effects were found in the ability of the interventions to change participants' weight attitudes, as well. Only four studies demonstrated some effectiveness in reducing negative weight attitudes. Swift et al.'s (2013) video-based intervention with medical students showed a significant reduction in explicit anti-fat attitudes that was maintained 6 weeks later. Brochu's (2020) intervention with clinical psychology trainees led to weaker endorsement of anti-fat attitudes and negative attitudes toward fat patients, and O'Brien et al.'s (2010) intervention with preservice health students led to less negative implicit attitudes toward fat people. Rukavina et al. (2010) showed that their intervention reduced kinesiology pre-professionals' social/character disparagement of fat people. It is important to note, however, that this prejudice reduction was not observed in Rukavina et al.'s (2008) study that used a similar intervention. Other studies also did not observe reductions in the endorsement of anti-fat attitudes. For example, Wijayatunga et al.'s (2019) intervention with kinesiology pre-professionals did not change participants' reports of social/character disparagement of fat people, nor their implicit weight attitudes. However, Wijayatunga et al. (2019) reported that implicit attitudes toward fat people worsened during the 1-month follow-up among students in the control condition, suggesting that the intervention may have protected against this worsening of implicit weight attitudes. Finally, Jones and Forhan (2019) found that physiotherapists' reports of anti-fat attitudes worsened after their 1-day workshop. That is, physiotherapists' attitudes toward fat people became more negative after the workshop, despite there being a reduction in their weight-control beliefs. Thus, as with weight stereotypes, some studies that were effective in reducing participants' beliefs regarding the controllability of weight were also effective in reducing participants' endorsement of negative weight attitudes, but others were not.

Cultural value of fatness

How may educators understand these mixed outcomes of controllability interventions that take place in health care training settings? From the perspective of the attribution-value model of prejudice, one possibility is to understand the cultural value of fatness that is communicated to the learning audience through the intervention. Of the 10 controllability interventions that are the focus of this analysis, nine of them reinforced a negative cultural value of fatness.

A negative cultural value of fatness was transmitted through these interventions via the dominant weight-normative paradigm of health that emphasizes the prevalence of fatness and its consequences on mortality and morbidity, as well as the perceived importance of weight loss for improved health outcomes. For example, in Wijayatunga et al.'s (2019) intervention, kinesiology undergraduate students first learned about body mass index (BMI) and how it correlated with health outcomes, including years of life lost, while the lecture later highlighted the complexity of fatness and dispelled myths that food causes fatness. Similarly, even though Wiese et al. (1992) presented medical students with non-stereotypical, positive portrayals of fat people and information that challenged weight stereotypes, they described fatness as a "handicap" and focused on the prevalence and health risk associated with fatness. The prevalence and consequences of fatness were also introduced to preservice health students in O'Brien et al.'s (2010) intervention. The videos on weight bias developed by the Rudd Center that were used by Swift et al. (2013) and Poutschi et al. (2013) also came from a perspective centered on the so-called "obesity epidemic," focusing on behavioral and lifestyle changes for weight loss while also acknowledging uncontrollable reasons for weight gain and a heavier weight status.

As further indications of a weight-normative perspective underlying these interventions, Persky and Eccleston (2011) and Jones and Forhan (2019) framed fatness as a disease and a risk factor for negative health outcomes. Although well-intentioned in their efforts, Rukavina et al. (2008, 2010) reinforced weight stereotypes in their intervention while attempting to persuade kinesiology pre-professionals to not blame fat people for their weight. In describing their intervention, they state: "Blame is not on the clients/students because they lack knowledge on the importance of healthy lifestyle, how to eat right or exercise appropriately, have low self-esteem and experience lots of barriers to becoming physically active" (Rukavina et al., 2008, p. 99). Thus, although intended to reduce weight bias, these interventions were guided by a weight-normative approach to health that views fatness negatively, and associates higher weight with ignorance, lack of intelligence, and poor health; they reinforced a negative cultural value of fatness.

What do controllability interventions that do not transmit a negative cultural value of fatness look like? Brochu (2020) was successful in designing such an intervention. Instead of situating fatness as a disease, advocating for weight loss, or focusing on the health consequences of fatness, the intervention challenged misconceptions regarding weight and health and emphasized the prevalence and harm of weight bias. Brochu (2020) incorporated critical weight science into an educational intervention for clinical psychology trainees that challenged assumptions underlying the dominant weight-normative approach to health. For example, participants learned that fatness is not necessarily unhealthy, that dieting is not effective for weight loss over the long-term, and that health behavior engagement can improve health among people of all sizes. Participants also learned about the pervasiveness of weight discrimination across a range of domains of daily living, the negative consequences of weight stigma and discrimination on physical health and psychological well-being, and weight-inclusive models of health such as Health at Every Size (HAES™).

Recommendations

The attribution-value model of prejudice highlights one way for fat pedagogy to be incorporated into health care training programs, by focusing on addressing weight controllability beliefs in conjunction with challenging the negative cultural value of fatness (Brochu, 2020). The incorporation of fat pedagogy into health care training is an important endeavor for at least three reasons. First, weight bias is pervasive in health care settings and among health care professionals and trainees, just as it is in broader society (Brochu et al., 2018; Pearl, 2018; Phelan et al., 2015). Second, despite its pervasiveness, weight bias is not addressed in health care training programs; training in multicultural and diversity issues rarely includes body size or weight stigma, and when body size is discussed in health care training programs, it is frequently done so from an individualized and medicalized perspective (Bergen & Mollen, 2019; Kasardo, 2019; Rothblum & Gartrell, 2019; Russell-Mayhew et al., 2016). Third, weight bias is harmful; within health care settings, it has physical and psychological health consequences that affect patients, providers, and students (Brochu et al., 2018; Chrisler & Barney, 2017; Hunger et al., 2015; Nutter et al., 2019; Pearl, 2018; Phelan et al., 2015). Many weight stigma researchers, health care practitioners, and public health policy makers have identified the important role of education and training in the reduction of weight stigma and discrimination in health care settings (Bergen & Mollen, 2019; Brochu et al., 2018; Chrisler & Barney, 2017; Hunger et al., 2020; McHugh & Kasardo, 2012; Nutter et al., 2018; Pearl, 2018; Rothblum & Gartrell, 2019).

In addition to recommendations provided by others to incorporate fat pedagogy, critical weight science, and discussion of weight stigma into education and training (Bergen & Mollen, 2019; Brochu, 2018; Cameron & Russel, 2016; Chrisler, 2018; Nutter et al., 2018; Rothblum & Gartrell, 2019), the current critical analysis makes salient three primary recommendation areas that are guided by the attribution-value model of prejudice. First, it is important to review weight bias reduction interventions critically and consider what cultural value of fatness they portray to participants. Many of the weight bias reduction interventions that are implemented in health care training settings are weight-loss centered, focus on the prevalence and consequences of fatness, or frame fatness as a disease. Even though these interventions intend to reduce weight bias, they reinforce a negative cultural value of fatness. This limits the ability of these interventions to effectively reduce weight bias, as they are situated within a social context that stigmatizes weight. It is important to critically consider all weight bias reduction interventions in this way, not only controllability interventions. As such, this recommendation extends to other interventions, as well. For example, weight bias reduction interventions that focus on increasing empathy may lack efficacy depending on what cultural value of fatness the intervention transmits to participants. The broader social context of weight bias reduction interventions must be thoughtfully considered to understand what value of fatness it communicates.

Second, it is recommended that educators in health care settings teach and inform others about weight bias, critical weight science, and weight-inclusive models of health. One mechanism underlying weight bias is the belief that weight can be lost easily if one tries hard enough (Crandall, 1994). These beliefs about the controllability of weight reinforce negative weight attitudes and stereotypes, such as viewing fat people negatively, holding fat people responsible for their weight, blaming fat people for health problems they may experience, perceiving fat people as lazy and unmotivated, and, as a result, being less willing to work with fat patients because they are thought of as a waste of time. Weight controllability beliefs are modifiable and can be addressed through controllability interventions.

Through the incorporation of critical weight science into weight bias reduction interventions, stigmatizing assumptions about weight and health can be rigorously challenged. Critical weight science calls into question many of the assumptions underlying the dominant weight-normative perspective on health (Bacon & Aphramor, 2011). For example, weight is a relatively poor predictor of health. Fat people may be healthy, and thin people may be unhealthy (Tomiyama et al., 2016). Fat people may live longer than thin people, or just as long (Flegal et al., 2013). Furthermore, dieting is not effective for weight loss over the long-term.

The most common long-term outcome of dieting is weight gain, not weight loss or weight maintenance (Mann et al, 2007; Rothblum, 2018). Weight loss is not needed to improve health; health behavior engagement leads to health improvements regardless of weight loss (Tomiyama et al., 2013). In fact, dieting and weight cycling are much more likely to harm health (Mann et al., 2007; Rothblum, 2018). Incorporating critical weight science into health care education provides a foundation for challenging beliefs regarding the controllability of weight and the negative cultural value of fatness.

Weight-inclusive models of health such as HAES are supported by critical weight science (Bacon & Aphramor, 2011; Calogero et al., 2019; Hunger et al., 2020; Logel et al., 2015; Mensinger et al., 2016; Tylka et al., 2014). Weight-inclusive models of health seek to encourage body acceptance, support intuitive eating, promote active embodiment, and reduce weight bias. Introducing students to weight-inclusive health models, shifts focus from body weight and weight loss to health and well-being for people of all sizes. Discussion of weight-inclusive health approaches allows students to gain an understanding of fatness from a social justice perspective.

Finally, the third area of recommendation is for educators to conduct research on the weight bias interventions that they implement. There is a need to better understand how these interventions work, for whom these interventions are effective, and what the long-term potential of these interventions are (Alberga et al., 2016). Dissemination of research on educational interventions to reduce weight bias, along with provision of the training tools used to conduct these interventions, will increase the likelihood that weight bias training will be provided in a range of education settings. Health care educators have a powerful role to play in raising awareness, building social consensus that weight bias is not acceptable, and destigmatizing fatness.

References

Alberga, A. S., Pickering, B. J., Hayden, K. A., Ball, G. D. C., Edwards, A., Jelinksi, S., Nutter, S., Oddie, S., Sharma, A. M., & Russel-Mayhew, S. (2016). Weight bias reduction in health professionals: A systematic review. *Clinical Obesity*, 6, 175–188. https://doi.org/10.1111/cob.12147

Bacon, L., & Aphramor, A. (2011). Weight science: Evaluating the evidence for a paradigm shift. *Nutrition Journal*, 10, 9. https://doi.org/10.1186/1475-2891-10-9

Bergen, M., & Mollen, D. (2019). Teaching sizeism: Integrating size into multicultural education and clinical training. *Women & Therapy*, 42(1–2), 164–180. https://doi.org/10.1080/02703149.2018.1524065

Brochu, P. M. (2020). Testing the effectiveness of a weight bias educational intervention among clinical psychology trainees. Advance online publication. *Journal of Applied Social Psychology*. https://doi.org/10.1111/jasp.12653

Brochu, P. M., Pearl, R. L., & Simontacchi, L. A. (2018). Weight stigma and related social factors in psychological care. In S. Cassin, R. Hawa, & S. Sockalingham (Eds.), *Psychological care in severe obesity: A practical and integrated approach* (pp. 42–60). Cambridge University Press. https://doi.org/10.1017/9781108241687.004

Calogero, R. M., Tylka, T. L., Mensinger, J. L., Meadows, A., & Daníelsdóttir, S. (2019). Recognizing the fundamental right to be fat: A weight-inclusive approach to size acceptance and healing from sizeism. *Women & Therapy, 42*, 22–44. https://doi.org/10.1080/02703149.2018.1524067

Cameron, E., & Russell, C. (Eds.). (2016). *The fat pedagogy reader: Challenging weight-based oppression through critical education*. Peter Lang.

Chrisler, J. C. (2018). Teaching health psychology from a size-acceptance perspective. *Fat Studies, 7*(1), 33–43. https://doi.org/10.1080/21604851.2017.1360668

Chrisler, J. C., & Barney, A. (2017). Sizeism is a health hazard. *Fat Studies, 6*(1), 38–53. http://dx.doi.org/10.1080/21604851.2016.1213066

Crandall, C. S. (1994). Prejudice against fat people: Ideology and self-interest. *Journal of Personality and Social Psychology, 66*(5), 882–894. https://doi.org/10.1037/0022-3514.66.5.882

Crandall, C. S., D'Anello, S., Sakalli, N., Lazarus, E., Nejtardt, G. W., & Feather, N. T. (2001). An attribution-value model of prejudice: Anti-fat attitudes in six nations. *Personality and Social Psychology Bulletin, 27*(1), 30–37. https://doi.org/10.1177/0146167201271003

Crandall, C. S., & Martinez, R. (1996). Culture, ideology, and antifat attitudes. *Personality and Social Psychology Bulletin, 22*(1), 1165–1176. https://doi.org/10.1177/01461672962211007

Daníelsdóttir, S., O'Brien, K. S., & Ciao, A. (2010). Anti-fat prejudice reduction: A review of published studies. *Obesity Facts, 3*, 47–58. https://doi.org/10.1159/000277067

Flegal, K. M., Kit, B. K., Orpana, H., & Graubard, B. I. (2013). Association of all-cause mortality with overweight and obesity using standard body mass index categories: A systematic review and meta-analysis. *JAMA, 309*, 71–82. https://doi.org/10.1001/jama.2012.113905

Hunger, J. M., Major, B., Blodorn, A., & Miller, C. T. (2015). Weighed down by stigma: How weight-based social identity threat contributes to weight gain and poor health. *Social and Personality Psychology Compass, 9*(6), 255–268. https://doi.org/10.1111/spc3.12172

Hunger, J. M., Smith, J. P., & Tomiyama, A. J. (2020). An evidence-based rationale for adopting weight-inclusive health policy. *Social Issues and Policy Review, 14*(1), 73–107. https://doi.org/10.1111/sipr.12062

Jones, C. A., & Forhan, M. (2019). Addressing weight bias and stigma of obesity amongst physiotherapists. Advance online publication. *Physiotherapy Theory and Practice*. https://doi.org/10.1080/09593985.2019.1648623

Kasardo, A. E. (2019). Size as diversity absent from multicultural textbooks. *Women & Therapy, 42*(1–2), 181–190. https://doi.org/10.1080/02703149.2018.1524069

Lee, M., Ata, R. N., & Brannick, M. T. (2014). Malleability of weight-biased attitudes and beliefs: A meta-analysis of weight bias reduction interventions. *Body Image, 11*, 251–259. https://doi.org/10.1016/j.bodyim.2014.03.003

Lippa, N. C., & Sanderson, S. C. (2012). Impact of information about obesity genomics on the stigmatization of overweight individuals: An experimental study. *Obesity, 20*, 2367–2376. https://doi.org/10.1038/oby.2012.144

Logel, C., Stinson, D. A., & Brochu, P. M. (2015). Weight loss is not the answer: A well-being solution to the "obesity problem." *Social and Personality Psychology Compass, 9*, 678–695. https://doi.org/10.1111/spc3.12223

Mann, T., Tomiyama, A. J., Westling, E., Lew, A.-M., Samuels, B., & Chatman, J. (2007). Medicare's search for effective obesity treatments: Diets are not the answer. *American Psychologist, 62*, 220–233. https://doi.org/10.1037/0003-066X.62.3.220

McHugh, M. C., & Kasardo, A. E. (2012). Anti-fat prejudice: The role of psychology in explication, education and eradication. *Sex Roles, 66*, 617–627. https://doi.org/10.1007/s11199-011-0099-x

Mensinger, J. L., Calogero, R. M., Stranges, S., & Tylka, T. L. (2016). A weight-neutral versus weight-loss approach for health promotion in women with high BMI: A randomized-control trial. *Appetite, 105*, 364–374. https://doi.org/10.1016/j.appet.2016.06.006

Nutter, S., Ireland, A., Alberga, A. S., Brun, I., Lefebvre, D., Hayden, K. A., & Russell-Mayhew, S. (2019). Weight bias in educational settings: A systematic review. *Current Obesity Reports, 8*, 185–200. https://doi.org/10.1007/s13679-019-00330-8

Nutter, S., Russell-Mayhew, S., Arthur, N., & Ellard, J. H. (2018). Weight bias and social justice: Implications for education and practice. *International Journal for the Advancement of Counselling, 40*(3), 213–226. https://doi.org/10.1007/s10447-018-9320-8

O'Brien, K. S., Puhl, R. M., Latner, J. D., Mir, A. S., & Hunter, J. A. (2010). Reducing anti-fat prejudice in preservice health students: A randomized trial. *Obesity, 18*, 2138–2144. https://doi.org/10.1038/oby.2010.79

Pearl, R. L. (2018). Weight bias and stigma: Public health implications and structural solutions. *Social Issues and Policy Review, 12*(1), 146–182. https://doi.org/10.1111/sipr.12043

Persky, S., & Eccleston, C. P. (2011). Impact of genetic causal information on medical students' clinical encounters with an obese virtual patient: Health promotion and social stigma. *Annals of Behavioral Medicine, 41*, 363–372. https://doi.org/10.1007/s12160-010-9242-0

Phelan, S. M., Burgess, D. J., Yeazel, M. W., Hellerstedt, W. L., Griffin, J. M., & van Ryn, M. (2015). Impact of weight bias and stigma on quality of care and outcomes for patients with obesity. *Obesity Reviews, 16*, 319–326. https://doi.org/10.1111/obr.12266

Poutschi, Y., Saks, N. S., Piasecki, A. K., Hahn, K. A., & Ferrante, J. M. (2013). Brief intervention effective in reducing weight bias in medical students. *Family Medicine, 45*(5), 345–348.

Rothblum, E. D. (2018). Slim chance for permanent weight loss. *Archives of Scientific Psychology, 6*, 63–69. https://doi.org/10.1037/arc0000043

Rothblum, E. D., & Gartrell, N. K. (2019). Sizeism in mental health training and supervision. *Women & Therapy, 42*(1–2), 147–155. https://doi.org/10.1080/02703149.2018.1524074

Rukavina, P. B., Li, W., & Rowell, M. B. (2008). A service learning based intervention to change attitudes toward obese individuals in kinesiology pre-professionals. *Social Psychology of Education, 11*, 95–112. https://doi.org/10.1007/s11218-007-9039-6

Rukavina, P. B., Li, W., Shen, B., & Sun, H. (2010). A service learning based project to change implicit and explicit bias toward obese individuals in kinesiology pre-professionals. *Obesity Facts, 3*, 117–126. https://doi.org/10.1159/000302794

Russell-Mayhew, S., Nutter, S., Alberga, A., Jelinksi, S., Ball, G. D. C., Edwards, A., Oddie, S., Sharma, A. M., Pickering, B., & Forhan, M. (2016). Environmental scan of weight bias exposure in primary health care training programs. *Canadian Journal for the Scholarship of Teaching and Learning, 7*(2), 5. https://doi.org/10.5206/cjsotl-rcacea.2016.2.5

Swift, J. A., Tischler, V., Markham, S., Gunning, I., Glazebrook, C., Beer, C., & Puhl, R. (2013). Are anti-stigma films a useful strategy for reducing weight bias among trainee healthcare professionals? Results of a pilot randomized control trial. *Obesity Facts, 6*, 91–102. https://doi.org/10.1159/000348714

Teachman, B. A., Gapinski, K. D., Brownell, K. D., Rawlins, M., & Jeyaram, S. (2003). Demonstrations of implicit anti-fat bias: The impact of providing causal information and evoking empathy. *Health Psychology, 22*(1), 68–78. https://doi.org/10.1037/0278-6133.22.1.68

Tomiyama, A. J., Ahlstrom, B., & Mann, T. (2013). Long-term effects of dieting: Is weight loss related to health? *Social and Personality Psychology Compass, 7,* 861–877. https://doi.org/10.1111/spc3.12076

Tomiyama, A. J., Hunger, J. M., Nguyen-Cuu, J., & Wells, C. (2016). Misclassification of cardiometabolic health when using body mass index categories in NHANES 2005-2012. *International Journal of Obesity, 40,* 883–886. https://doi.org/10.1038/ijo.2016.17

Tylka, T. L., Annunziato, R. A., Burgard, D., Daníelsdóttir, S., Shuman, E., Davis, C., & Calogero, R. M. (2014). The weight-inclusive versus weight-normative approach to health: Evaluating the evidence for prioritizing well-being over weight loss. *Journal of Obesity, 2014,* 983495. https://doi.org/10.1155/2014/983495

University of Connecticut Rudd Center for Food Policy & Obesity. (2009a). *Weight prejudice: Myths & facts* [Video]. http://www.uconnruddcenter.org/weight-bias-stigma-videos-exposing-weight-bias

University of Connecticut Rudd Center for Food Policy & Obesity. (2009b). *Weight bias in health care* [Video]. http://www.uconnruddcenter.org/weight-bias-stigma-videos-exposing-weight-bias

Weiner, B. (1995). Responsibility and stigmatization. In *Judgments of responsibility: A foundation for a theory of social conduct* (pp. 53–86). Guilford Press.

Weiner, B., Perry, R. P., & Magnusson, J. (1988). An attributional analysis of reactions to stigmas. *Journal of Personality and Social Psychology, 55*(5), 738–748. https://doi.org/10.1037/0022-3514.55.5.738

Wiese, H. J. C., Wilson, J. F., Jones, R. A., & Neises, M. (1992). Obesity stigma reduction in medical students. *International Journal of Obesity, 16,* 859–868.

Wijayatunga, N. N., Kim, Y., Butsch, W. S., & Dhurandhar, E. J. (2019). The effects of a teaching intervention on weight bias among kinesiology undergraduate students. *International Journal of Obesity, 43,* 2273–2281. https://doi.org/10.1038/s41366-019-0325-0

15 Conclusion

A call to fatten pedagogy because lives depend on it

Heather A. Brown and Nancy Ellis-Ordway

Ellen Maud Bennett, a resident of Victoria, British Columbia, died at age 64. A smart, creative woman, Ellen worked for stage and screen. Even though the picture that accompanies her death notice was taken just days before her passing, you can see that she is funny and full of life. Her official cause of death was inoperable cancer, but that is not the entire story.

According to her obituary, Ellen Maud Bennett was a victim of weight bias and medical fatphobia.

> A final message Ellen wanted to share was about the fat shaming she endured from the medical profession. Over the past few years of feeling unwell she sought out medical intervention and no one offered any support or suggestions beyond weight loss. Ellen's dying wish was that women of size make her death matter by advocating strongly for their health and not accepting that fat is the only relevant health issue. (Obituary of Ellen Maud Bennett, 2018, n.p.)

Far too many fat individuals live with the knowledge that they, too, could be Ellen Maud Bennett—ignored or maligned because of their weight, with the only preventative care or medical intervention provided a prescription to "lose weight," a prescription that fails nearly all the time. Due to a weight-loss-first approach to health care for fat people and the weight bias and discrimination that often drive or accompany that approach, fat individuals avoid seeking care (Amy et al., 2006; Drury & Louis, 2002; Hunger et al., 2015; Phelan et al., 2015), including but not limited to cancer screenings (Aldrich & Hackley, 2010; Cohen et al., 2008; Fontaine et al., 1998; Rosen & Schneider, 2004). Weight bias can also actually cause poor physical and mental health and poor health behaviors (Brown, 2012; Carr et al., 2007; Dickerson & Kemeny, 2004; Faith et al., 2002; Himmelstein et al., 2015; Hunger et al., 2015; Major et al., 2012; Matthews et al., 2005; Pearl et al., 2015; Schvey et al., 2014; Sutin et al., 2014; Tomiyama et al., 2015).

In a blog post, Linda (aka Fluffy Kitten Party), brings the lived experience of medical fatphobia to vivid life:

DOI: 10.4324/9781003057000-17

It's chairs you can't fit into, it's doctors complaining about your body *to you* like you should apologize for making their day hard, it's medical equipment that's not built for you so it's harder (if not impossible) to get diagnosed and treated, it's having to trust people to take care of you when you're unconscious and vulnerable when they have been openly hostile to you, it's being told you can't have surgery you need because anesthesia is too risky but then the anesthesia suddenly not being a problem if you let them amputate part of your stomach. (Fluffy Kitten Party, 2021, para. 14)

Weight bias and medical fatphobia can and do kill fat people. This realistic fear has become even more palpable and immediate during COVID-19. Not only has weight stigma and fat shaming increased during quarantine during the pandemic (see Kumar's 2020 article "Shelter in place does not mean shelter on the couch" as an example), but experiences with prior medical fatphobia and weight bias could be leading fat individuals to avoid medical care even for COVID-19. Le Brocq et al. (2020) reported that the "people living with obesity" with whom they work in the United Kingdom expressed "genuine, all-consuming fears of contracting COVID-19" (para. 3) with many of their patients convinced they would not be provided with appropriate and needed medical care. Sultan (2021) also reported that fat individuals in the United States expressed the same fears—and that the fear could cause them to not seek out medical care until it is too late.

Avoidance of health care professionals should be an important critique of any research on the connections between weight and COVID-19 outcomes. Despite media insistence that "obesity" is a risk factor for contracting and dying from COVID-19, the data show a different story. For example, Sun et al. (2016) found that poor outcomes for fat individuals during the H1N1 epidemic were connected not to weight per se but rather to doctors not prescribing early antiviral treatments to larger individuals. A similar situation is occurring with COVID-19 (Harrison, 2020). According to Harrison, the studies that have a reported a correlation between "obesity" and poor COVID-19 outcomes also are flawed in many ways, including not controlling for the social determinants of health such as racism, access to health care, poverty, and—yes—weight bias and discrimination. "There has been an open debate about whether fat people are worth giving ventilators to, and I don't think we think enough about the impact of hearing the worth of your life debated in public" (Gordon, 2021, as cited in Sole-Smith, 2021, para. 5).

Do no harm

As you have read the chapters of this book, it should be increasingly clear that weight stigma and bias create ethical questions for practitioners in all medical fields. While codes of ethics differ among professional groups, we have certain values in common such as enhancing quality of life, respecting human dignity and diversity, and promoting social justice (Academy of Nutrition and Dietetics, 2018; American Counseling Association, 2014; American Nurses Association, 2015; American Psychological Association, 2017; American Public Health Association, 2019; National Association of Social Workers, 2017; Riddick, 2003). Overarching principles include beneficence/non-maleficence, or "do no harm," self-determination/autonomy, informed consent, evidence-based practice, competence, conflicts of interest, and social justice.

"Do no harm" may not be as clear cut as it seems. Weight stigma clearly results in harm when it interferes with access to care, when it creates shame, and when it is the basis for oppression and discrimination (Abu-Odeh, 2014). The hierarchy inherent in the medical professional/patient relationship creates an inequality in power, meaning that we, as the professional, have a responsibility to use that power differential in the best interest of the patient. When we recommend weight loss, we are causing harm.

Self-determination, autonomy, and informed consent are intertwined. Our patients deserve the opportunity to make decisions for themselves and for their care, but they also deserve complete information necessary for making choices. When we receive something as simple as a flu shot, we must indicate by our signature that we understand all of the possible risks, even the unlikely ones. Yet recommendations for weight loss are not accompanied by thorough explanations of the high rates of failure or the possible negative outcomes for physical and mental health.

One of the arguments for focusing on weight loss is "It is what the patient asks for." However, when we recommend an intervention with a high failure rate and numerous negative side effects because it is what they want to hear, we are not providing patient-centered care (Bianchi & Ricupero, 2020). Physicians do not prescribe addictive or dangerous medicines just because the patient asks for it, and therapists don't provide "conversion therapy" just because a patient asks for it. It is our responsibility to ensure that patients are properly informed of benefits and risks and that they know they can make decisions without coercion, duress, or undue influence (Olson & Stokes, 2016). Autonomy and self-determination require informed consent, which requires accurate, transparent, understandable information (Bianchi & Ricupero, 2020).

When patients come to us for care, they assume that our recommendations and interventions will be evidence based. The evidence supporting weight loss for health is questionable and the evidence for sustainable weight loss is entirely lacking. The evidence that weight bias negatively affects health, access to health care, and quality of life is considerable and growing. As clinicians, researchers, and educators, we are responsible for focusing on well-supported evidence. Additionally, we must continuously educate ourselves and change our practice when new evidence suggests new practice.

We also can increase our competence by reviewing all of the information available while being very aware of our own biases and preconceived ideas. Implicit weight bias permeates our culture, and it is understandable that we are all affected by it. It is essential that we are aware of this in our own practices as well as in our education. The lucrative dieting industry influences research publications and general media. Conflicts of interest can be subtle, such as research that is funded by a company making weight loss drugs, or more obvious, such as clinicians who benefit financially from weight loss surgeries or diet programs.

Respect for the dignity and worth of the individual is inherent in all of the work that we do. When stigma of any kind interferes, what is our responsibility? Social inequality plays a large role in health, for both individuals and the community. Stigma erodes dignity, leading to discrimination and inequality (Bayer, 2008). When we advocate for social change, we improve the landscape for everyone. When we challenge weight stigma in ourselves, our practices, our colleagues, our training, and our communities, we all benefit. Our codes of ethics include social justice as a principle because it is the right thing to do. "The use of stigma perpetuates and produces injustice and is therefore unethical" (Abu-Odeh, 2014, p. 260).

Social determinants, such as poverty, discrimination, access to education and health care, pollution, and the built environment, have a greater impact on health than individual behaviors (Centers for Disease Control and Prevention, n.d.). However, changing social determinants is complicated and costly, requiring a shifting focus as well as political will. A focus on changing an individual's body size is much simpler but is a distraction from larger issues that are more challenging to address. Programs focusing on "the obesity epidemic" by targeting individual behavior and responsibility then reinforce and maintain the status quo.

There is acknowledgement, at least, among a majority of health care professions that bias against fat individuals is problematic. Many researchers, educators, and practitioners have started the work of trying to address weight bias and discrimination among current and future health care providers. This work, however, is still grounded in a weight-loss approach. Fatness is still unhealthy, still a diseased state, and doctors and fat people must, within this system, battle to end fatness. Such an approach reinforces the very bias against fat individuals that we address here.

This work

This collection is only the start of the work to tackle that harmful status quo. In these chapters, our authors—practitioners, educators, and students, family, friends, and fat individuals—address issues of weight bias and fatphobia within health care professions and explore ways to address those issues without further harming fat individuals—or demand that they lose weight before being deemed worthy of medical treatment. We believe this collection represents a foundational but critically important step toward the very basic principle that all health care professionals should embrace but rarely do when it comes to fat individuals: do no harm. It is time for our medical professionals to treat fat people like people.

We also acknowledge that this work is not perfect nor is it fully complete. While issues of race, class, gender, sexuality, socioeconomic status, and other aspects of identity and the social determinants of health are addressed and wrestled with by the authors in the collection, the field remains overwhelmingly White, female dominated, and cishet. Fat BIPOC and fat queer/trans individuals still face additional barriers to health care access and dignity in treatment that need to be explored in specific detail and in more depth than these chapters do.

What we have collected here represents work that:

> ... doesn't need to be perfect. It doesn't need to fix everything in one fell swoop. It can be baby steps like getting more accessible seating in doctor's offices, along with the long-term work of educating medical professionals about weight stigma, advocating for fat bodies to be studied more (because at the moment we are rarely studied beyond measuring our deviance from "normal"), building a health care system with doctors who are not befuddled by the sight of us and have equipment and resources to correctly diagnose and properly treat us, and making health care *truly* affordable and accessible to people of all stations. It's a mixture of small pragmatic changes and large endeavors that will require legislation, long-term sustained effort, and buy-in from people in power. It's going to require coalition-building and multipronged efforts from groups and movements with compatible, complimentary goals. *This is how social change works.* It's mundane and slow and beautiful and revolutionary all at once. And if you stack the small and medium-size and mundane accomplishments one on top of one another, you can use them to build something new. (Fluffy Kitten Party, 2021, para. 22)

Building something new

In her work in teaching about social change and weight bias, Nancy likes to remind participants that change does not happen immediately. Rather, she encourages each participant to imagine a large ocean vessel. Crossing the wide-open ocean, the vessel travels smoothly unless something impedes its progress. Once it arrives at dock, however, it becomes unwieldy. It cannot maneuver delicately to reach its ultimate destination—the pier. Instead, it needs help to make those small incremental moves that will allow it to dock successfully. That's where the tugboats come in—each tug pushing or pulling the larger vessel moment by moment, foot by foot, and—in the end—inch by inch, until the larger vessel is where it actually needs to be.

Each chapter in this book is its own tugboat in maneuvering current and future health care practitioners to where they need to actually go if their goal is to help rather than harm fat patients. Each chapter uncovers moments where health care providers are influenced by conscious or unconscious weight bias and discrimination, where medical associations declare "obesity" a disease against their own advisory council's evidence-based recommendations (Pittman, 2013), and instructors fail to call out problematic beliefs, behaviors, and practices in their students. Each chapter also provides potential solutions, grounded in pedagogy, that address weight bias in ways that do not cause further stigmatization of fat individuals. The goal of health care professions should be to support fat individuals in reaching their own self-determined goals, to listen to their needs and their own understandings about the bodies in which they live daily, and to treat fat individuals with dignity and respect. The goal should not be to find a better more compassionate way to tell fat individuals that they have no right to exist in their bodies as their bodies currently exist.

In 2020, Black medical students at the University of Pittsburgh School of Medicine wrote an addition to the Hippocratic oath to address racial injustice and the failures of the medical community to serve all people with the same access to care, dignity, and evidence-based practice. Their new oath includes the following:

> We recognize the fundamental failings of our health care and political systems in serving vulnerable communities. This oath is the first step in our enduring commitment to repairing the injustices against those historically ignored and abused in medicine: Black patients, Indigenous patients, Patients of Color and all marginalized populations who have received substandard care as a result of their identity and limited resources. (University of Pittsburgh School of Medicine's Class of 2024, 2020, para. 12)

Fat people have been ignored and abused in health care settings. As a result of bias and discrimination, fat individuals avoid seeking care and experience far worse health outcomes than others who are not ignored or abused by systemic medical fatphobia. Current and future health care professionals must learn new ways to treat fat individuals outside of the dominant "obesity" paradigm.

Change has started and change will continue—perhaps not as quickly as all of us would like. But the change must continue—because lives depend on it.

References

Abu-Odeh, D. (2014). Fat stigma and public health: A theoretical framework and ethical analysis. *Kennedy Institute of Ethics Journal, 24*(3), 247–265. https://doi.org/10.1353/ken.2014.0024

Academy of Nutrition and Dietetics. (2018). *Code of ethics for the nutrition and dietetics profession.* Commission on Dietetic Registration. https://homeworkhandlers.com/code-of-ethics-for-the-nutrition-and-dietetics-profession/#:~:text=%20Code%20of%20Ethics%20for%20the%20Nutrition%20and,Professionalism%20%28Beneficence%29%20Nutrition%20and%20dietetics%20practitioners...%20More%20

Aldrich, T., & Hackley, B. (2010). The impact of obesity on gynecologic cancer screening: An integrative literature review. *Journal of Midwifery & Women's Health, 55*(4), 344–356. https://doi.org/10.1016/j.jmwh.2009.10.001

American Counseling Association. (2014). *ACA code of ethics.* https://www.counseling.org/resources/aca-code-of-ethics.pdf

American Nurses Association (2015). *Code of ethics for nurses with interpretive statements.* https://homecaremissouri.org/mahc/documents/CodeofEthicswInterpretive Statements20141.pdf#:~:text=The%20Code%20of%20Ethics%20for%20Nurses%20 with%20Interpretive,process%20of%20revision%20by%20the%20American%20 Nurses%20Association

American Psychological Association. (2017). *Ethical principles of psychologists and code of conduct* (2002, amended effective June 1, 2010, and January 1, 2017). http://www.apa. org/ethics/code/index.html

American Public Health Association. (2019). *Public health code of ethics.* http://ethics. iit.edu/ecodes/node/4734#:~:text=A%20code%20of%20ethics%20for%20public%20 health%20clarifies,of%20the%20public%20health%20institutions%20that%20 serve%20them

Amy, N. K., Aalborg, A., Lyons, P., & Keranen, L. (2006). Barriers to routine gyneco- logical cancer screening for White and African-American obese women. *International Journal of Obesity, 30*(1), 147–155. https://doi.org/10.1038/sj.ijo.0803105

Bayer, R. (2008). Stigma and the ethics of public health: Not can we but should we. *Social Science & Medicine, 67*(3), 463–472. https://doi.org/10.1016/j.socscimed.2008.03.017

Bianchi, A., & Ricupero, M. (2020). Questioning the ethics of promoting weight loss in clin- ical practice. *Canadian Journal of Bioethics, 3*(1), 95. https://doi.org/10.7202/1070228ar

Brown, H. (2012). *Fashioning a self from which to thrive: Negotiating size privilege as a fat woman learner at a small liberal arts college in the Midwest* (Doctoral dissertation). DeKalb, IL: Northern Illinois University.

Carr, D., Friedman, M. A., & Jaffe, K. (2007). Understanding the relationship between obesity and positive and negative affect: The role of psychosocial mechanisms. *Body Image, 4*(2), 165–177. https://doi.org/10.1016/j.bodyim.2007.02.004

Centers for Disease Control and Prevention. (n.d.). *Social determinants of health.* https:// www.cdc.gov/nchhstp/socialdeterminants/index.html

Cohen, S. S., Palmieri, R. T., Nyante, S. J., Koralek, D. O., Kim, S., Bradshaw, P., & Olshan, A. F. (2008). A review: Obesity and screening for breast, cervical, and colorec- tal cancer in women. *Cancer, 112*(9), 1892–1904. https://doi.org/10.1002/cncr.23408

Dickerson, S. S., & Kemeny, M. E. (2004). Acute stressors and cortisol responses: A the- oretical integration and synthesis of laboratory research. *Psychological Bulletin, 130*(3), 355. https://psycnet.apa.org/doi/10.1037/0033-2909.130.3.355

Drury, C. A., & Louis, M. (2002). Exploring the association between body weight, stigma of obesity, and health care avoidance. *Journal of the American Academy of Nurse Practitioners, 14*(12), 554–561. https://doi.org/10.1111/j.1745-7599.2002.tb00089.x

Faith, M. S., Leone, M. A., Ayers, T. S., Heo, M., & Pietrobelli, A. (2002). Weight crit- icism during physical activity, coping skills, and reported physical activity in children. *Pediatrics, 110*(2), e23–e23. https://doi.org/10.1542/peds.110.2.e23

Fluffy Kitten Party. (2021, February 11). *A plea.* https://fluffykittenparty.com/2021/ 02/11/a-plea/?fbclid=IwAR0-Dj5dYKewIrGWcaWiiDcqGYO4N3myUn8G0E5Sx1a YRy47z8yh9YZfSJI

Fontaine, K. R., Faith, M. S., Allison, D. B., & Cheskin, L. J. (1998). Body weight and health care among women in the general population. *Archives of Family Medicine, 7*(4), 381.

Harrison, C. (2020, April 7). COVID-19 does not discriminate by body weight. *Wired.* https://www.wired.com/story/covid-19-does-not-discriminate-by-body-weight/

Himmelstein, M. S., Incollingo Belsky, A. C., & Tomiyama, A. J. (2015). The weight of stigma: Cortisol reactivity to manipulated weight stigma. *Obesity, 23*(2), 368–374. https://doi.org/10.1002/oby.20959

Hunger, J. M., Major, B., Blodorn, A., & Miller, C. T. (2015). Weighed down by stigma: How weight-based social identity threat contributes to weight gain and poor health. *Social and Personality Psychology Compass*, 9(6), 255–268. https://doi.org/10.1111/spc3.12172

Kumar, V. (2020, April 9). Shelter in place does not mean shelter on the couch: How to stay healthy when COVID-19 sheltering. *ABCNews*. https://abcnews.go.com/Health/shelter-place-shelter-couch-stay-healthy-covid-19/story?id=69963756

Le Brocq, S., Clare, K., Bryant, M., Roberts, K., & Tahrani, A. A. (2020). Obesity and COVID-19: A call for action from people living with obesity. *The Lancet Diabetes & Endocrinology*, 8(8), 652–654. https://doi.org/10.1016/S2213-8587(20)30236-9

National Association of Social Workers. (2017). *Code of ethics of the National Association of Social Workers.* https://naswor.socialworkers.org/Membership/Resources/Code-of-Ethics

Major, B., Eliezer, D., & Rieck, H. (2012). The psychological weight of weight stigma. *Social Psychological and Personality Science*, 3(6), 651–658. https://doi.org/10.1177%2F1948550611434400

Matthews, K. A., Salomon, K., Kenyon, K., & Zhou, F. (2005). Unfair treatment, discrimination, and ambulatory blood pressure in Black and White adolescents. *Health Psychology*, 24(3), 258. https://psycnet.apa.org/doi/10.1037/0278-6133.24.3.258

Obituary of Ellen Maud Bennett. (2018). *Legacy.* https://www.legacy.com/amp/obituaries/timescolonist/189588876?fbclid=IwAR0-Dj5dYKewIrGWcaWiiDcqGYO4N3myUn8G0E5Sx1aYRy47z8yh9YZfSJI

Olson, L. L., & Stokes, F. (2016). The ANA code of ethics for nurses with interpretive statements: Resource for nursing regulation. *Journal of Nursing Regulation*, 7(2), 9–20. https://doi.org/10.1016/s2155-8256(16)31073-0

Pearl, R. L., Puhl, R. M., & Dovidio, J. F. (2015). Differential effects of weight bias experiences and internalization on exercise among women with overweight and obesity. *Journal of Health Psychology*, 20(12), 1626–1632. https://doi.org/10.1177%2F1359105313520338

Phelan, S. M., Burgess, D. J., Yeazel, M. W., Hellerstedt, W. L., Griffin, J. M., & van Ryn, M. (2015). Impact of weight bias and stigma on quality of care and outcomes for patients with obesity. *Obesity Reviews*, 16(4), 319–326. https://doi.org/10.1111/obr.12266

Pittman, D. (2013). AMA house votes against council, calls obesity a disease. *MedPage Today*. https://www.medpagetoday.com/meetingcoverage/ama/39952

Riddick, F. A. (2003). The code of medical ethics of the American Medical Association. *The Ochsner Journal*, 5(2), 6–10.

Rosen, A. B., & Schneider, E. C. (2004). Colorectal cancer screening disparities related to obesity and gender. *Journal of General Internal Medicine*, 19(4), 332–338. https://doi.org/10.1111/j.1525-1497.2004.30339.x

Schvey, N. A., Puhl, R. M., & Brownell, K. D. (2014). The stress of stigma: Exploring the effect of weight stigma on cortisol reactivity. *Psychosomatic Medicine*, 76(2), 156–162. https://doi.org/10.1097/PSY.0000000000000031

Sole-Smith, V. (2021, January 11). How fatphobia is leading to poor care in the pandemic: Weight stigma in health care can impact the care people get for COVID-19. *Elemental/Medium.* https://elemental.medium.com/how-fatphobia-is-leading-to-poor-care-in-the-pandemic-1b594682704

Sultan, R. (2021, February 26). Here's how it feels to be "fat enough" to get the COVID vaccine. *InStyle.* https://www.instyle.com/beauty/health-fitness/bmi-vaccine-covid-eligibility-fatphobia-medicine?fbclid=IwAR1o_-H5XbIuU_IYPbPhqOX5wClP6EXhIMOKIV7U6vm693YJC3kJDWTeiME

Sun, Y., Wang, Q., Yang, G., Lin, C., Zhang, Y., & Yang, P. (2016). Weight and prognosis for influenza A (H1N1) pdm09 infection during the pandemic period between 2009 and 2011: A systematic review of observational studies with meta-analysis. *Infectious Diseases*, *48*(11–12), 813–822. https://doi.org/10.1080/23744235.2016.1201721

Sutin, A. R., Stephan, Y., Luchetti, M., & Terracciano, A. (2014). Perceived weight discrimination and C-reactive protein. *Obesity*, *22*(9), 1959–1961. https://doi.org/10.1002/oby.20789

Tomiyama, A. J., Finch, L. E., Belsky, A. C. I., Buss, J., Finley, C., Schwartz, M. B., & Daubenmier, J. (2015). Weight bias in 2001 versus 2013: Contradictory attitudes among obesity researchers and health professionals. *Obesity*, *23*(1), 46–53. https://doi.org/10.1002/oby.20910

University of Pittsburgh School of Medicine's Class of 2024. (2020). *Modern-day Hippocrates: Incoming school of medicine students write their own oath*. PittWire. https://www.pittwire.pitt.edu/news/modern-day-hippocrates-incoming-school-medicine-students-write-their-own-oath

Index

Printed in the United States
by Baker & Taylor Publisher Services